ENVIRONMENTAL TOXICOLOGY

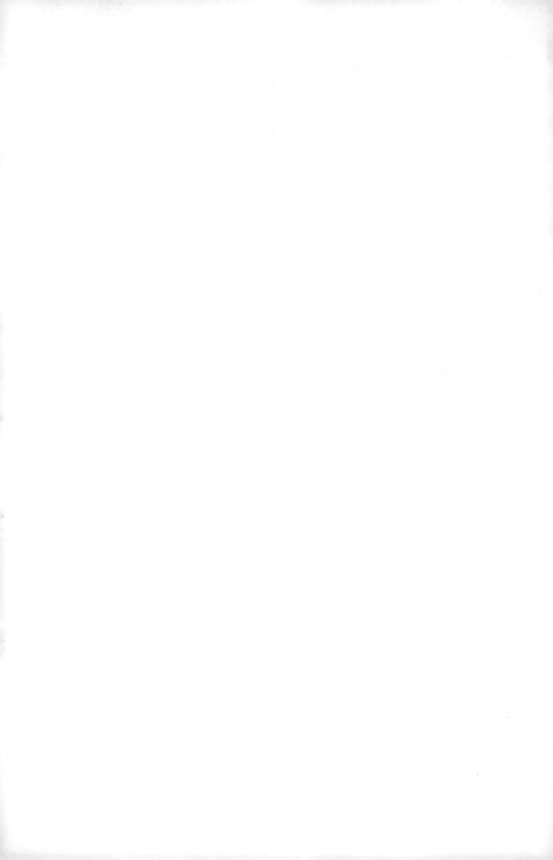

ENVIRONMENTAL TOXICOLOGY

Principles and Policies

Edited by

SATU M. SOMANI, Ph.D.

Associate Professor of Pharmacology and Toxicology
Department of Pharmacology
Southern Illinois University
School of Medicine
Springfield, Illinois

and

FINIS L. CAVENDER, Ph.D.

Director, Inhalation Toxicology
ToxiGenics
Decatur, Illinois

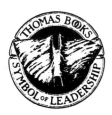

CHARLES C THOMAS • PUBLISHER
Springfield • Illinois • U.S.A.

Published and Distributed Throughout the World by
CHARLES C THOMAS • PUBLISHER
2600 South First Street
Springfield, Illinois, 62717, U.S.A.

© *1981, by* CHARLES C THOMAS • PUBLISHER
ISBN 0-398-04549-6
Library of Congress Catalog Card Number: 81-8936

*With THOMAS BOOKS careful attention is given to all details
of manufacturing and design. It is the Publisher's desire to
present books that are satisfactory as to their physical qualities
and artistic possibilities and appropriate for their particular use.
THOMAS BOOKS will be true to those laws of quality that
assure a good name and good will.*

Library of Congress Cataloging in Publication Data
Main entry under title:
Environmental toxicology, principles, and policies.

　　Based on a symposium organized by the Decatur/
Springfield Section of the American Chemical Society.
　　Bibliography: p.
　　Includes index.
　　1. Toxicology—Congresses. 2. Pollution—Toxicology
—Congresses. I. Somani, Satu M.
II. Cavender, Finis L. III. American Chemical Society.
Decatur/Springfield Section.
RA1191.E58　　　　615.9　　　　81-8936
ISBN 0-398-04549-6　　　　　　　AACR2

Printed in the United States of America
SC-R-1

CONTRIBUTORS

MICHAEL ALAVANJA, Dr. P.H.
Senior Epidemiologist
Division of Criteria Documentation and
  Standards Development
National Institute for Occupational Safety
  and Health
5600 Fishers Lane
Rockville, MD 20857

ROGER E. BEYLER
Department of Chemistry and Biochemistry
Southern Illinois University
Carbondale, IL 62901

W. M. BUSEY, D.V.M., Ph.D.
Experimental Pathology Laboratories, Inc.
P.O. Box 474
Herndon, VA 22070

FINIS L. CAVENDER, Ph.D.
Director, Inhalation Toxicology
ToxiGenics, Inc.
1800 East Pershing Road
Decatur, IL 62526

BEVERLY Y. COCKRELL, D.V.M., Ph.D.
Electron Microscopist/Pathologist
Experimental Pathology Laboratories, Inc.
P.O. Box 474
Herndon, VA 22070

JOSEPH A. COTRUVO, Ph.D.
Director, Standards and Criteria
Environmental Protection Agency
401 M. Street, S.W.
Washington, D.C. 20406

MILTON HEJTMANCIK, Jr., Ph.D.
Department of Pharmacology
Southern Illinois University
School of Medicine
801 N. Rutledge
Springfield, IL 62708

DEAN M. HARTLEY
Institute of Environmental Studies
University of Illinois
1000 W. Western Avenue
Urbana, IL 61801

JAMES B. JOHNSTON, Ph.D.
Institute of Environmental Studies
University of Illinois
1000 W. Western Avenue
Urbana, IL 61801

MERYL H. KAROL, Ph.D.
Dept. Industrial Environmental Health
   Sciences
Graduate School of Public Health
University of Pittsburgh
Pittsburgh, PA 15261

MICHAEL P. MAUZY, Director
Illinois State Environmental Protection
   Agency
2200 Churchill Road
Springfield, IL 62706

VERA K. MEYERS, Ph.D.
Department of Chemistry and Biochemistry
Southern Illinois University
School of Medicine
Carbondale, IL 62901

RICHARD H. MOY, M.D.
Dean and Provost
Southern Illinois University
School of Medicine
801 N. Rutledge
Springfield, IL 62708

MICHAEL J. PLEWA, Ph.D.
Environmental Research Laboratories
Institute for Environmental Studies
University of Illinois
1000 W. Western Avenue
Urbana, IL 61801

JOSEPH K. PRINCE
Regional Toxicologist/Health Efforts
  Specialist—Region V
U.S. Environmental Protection Agency
Water Supply Branch
230 South Dearborn Street
Chicago, IL 60604

SATU M. SOMANI, Ph.D.
Department of Pharmacology
Southern Illinois University
School of Medicine
801 N. Rutledge
Springfield, IL 62708

DAVID L. SWIFT, Ph.D.
Professor of Environmental Medicine
School of Medicine
Johns Hopkins University
615 N. Wolfe Street
Baltimore, MD 21205

JAMES B. TERRILL, Ph.D.
Environmental Health Laboratory
Monsanto Chemical Company
800 N. Lindberg
St. Louis, MO 63166

B. J. WILLIAMS
Department of Pharmacology and Toxicology
The University of Texas Medical Branch
Galveston, TX 77550

PREFACE

This appeared to be a particularly appropriate time for the Decatur/Springfield Section of the American Chemical Society to organize its first symposium on "Environmental Toxicology: Principles and Policies." It was gratifying to see the auditorium filled to capacity and the immense interest shown in the topics presented. The topics were varied and fascinating in themselves, but, because of time constraints, could not be developed fully. We hope that the papers presented in the symposium will contribute to a better understanding, both by scientists and the public, of the problems arising with environmental toxicology.

Ms. Karen Harlin, Chairperson of this Section of ACS, in her welcome speech, addressed the basis of the symposium.

> As scientist and consumers we are all concerned with a safe workplace, safe products and unpolluted sources of water to drink and air to breathe. But how do we determine what compounds are safe? Is a little exposure acceptable but is a large amount hazardous? Since it is impossible to achieve a no risk situation—at what risk level could we be reasonably safe and on what basis are Government regulations formed to promote this situation? Human epidemiological cancer studies relating incidence of cancer to exposure situations parallel results obtained from animal toxicity studies. What is toxic to man is also toxic to some other species of animal—but how do we design and interpret the results of these animal studies? Toxicity tests must be translated into meaningful results which can then form the basis for establishing guidelines for the handling, use, labeling, and disposal of chemicals in our environment.

This Section is grateful to the Organizing Committee members: Ed Acheson, Milikan University; Carl Niekamp, A. E. Staley Co.; Finis Cavender, ToxiGenics, Inc.; Satu Somani, Southern Illinois University; Gary Germann, Illinois EPA; Angela Tin, Southern Illinois University; and those volunteers who contributed so much of their time and effort to make this symposium successful.

A special thanks to Ms. Diana Smith of the Department of Pharmacology, Southern Illinois University and Ms. Linda Gardner of ToxiGenics for their valuable secretarial work and typing the manuscripts.

Finally, we sincerely thank every contributor who unselfishly and without honoraria presented their topics at the symposium.

SMS
FLC

INTRODUCTORY REMARKS

RICHARD H. MOY

I suppose all groups, when they get together, are assured that what they are doing is important, but to call the topic that you are considering important is an understatement. What I would like to do is to read to you from the "Prophets."

The tragedy of the commons develops in this way. Picture a pasture open to all. It is to be expected that each herdsman will try to keep as many cattle as possible on the commons. Such an arrangement may work reasonably satisfactorily for centuries because tribal wars, poaching, and disease keep the numbers of both man and beast well below the carrying capacity of the land. Finally, however, comes the day of reckoning, that is, the day when the long-desired goal of social stability becomes a reality. At this point the inherent logic of the commons remorselessly generates tragedy.

As a rational being, each herdsman seeks to maximize his gain. Explicitly or implicitly, more or less consciously, he asks, 'What is the utility to me of adding one more animal to my herd?' This utility has one negative and one positive component.

1. The positive component is a function of the increment of one animal. Since the herdsman receives all the proceeds from the sale of the additional animal, the positive utility is nearly +1.

2. The negative component is a function of the additional overgrazing created by one more animal. Since, however, the effects of overgrazing are shared by all the herdsmen, the negative utility for any particular decision-making herdsman is only a fraction of −1.

Adding together the component partial utilities, the rational herdsman concludes that the only sensible course for him to pursue is to add another animal to his herd. And another.... But this is the conclusion reached by each and every rational herdsman sharing a commons. Therein is the tragedy. Each man is locked into a system that compels him to increase his herd without limit—in a world that is limited. Ruin is the destination toward which all men rush, each pursuing his own best interest in a society that believes in the freedom of the commons. Freedom in a commons brings ruin to all.

In a reverse way, the tragedy of the commons appears in problems of pollution. Here it is not a question of taking something out of the commons, but of putting something in—sewage, or chemical, radioactive, and heat wastes into water; noxious and dangerous fumes into the air; and distracting and unpleasant advertising signs into the line of sight. The calculations of utility are much the same as before. The rational man finds that his share of the cost of the wastes he discharges into the commons is less than the cost of purifying his wastes before releasing them. Since this is true for everyone, we are locked into a system of 'fouling our own nest,' so long as we behave only as independent, rational, free enterprisers.

That, of course, is Garrett Hardin's essay of "Tragedy of the Commons."[1]

His was not the first voice. Albert Schweitzer said, "Man has lost his capacity to foresee and to forestall. He will end by destroying the earth."[2] E. B. White said, "I am pessimistic about the human race because it is too ingenious for its own good. Our approach to nature is to beat it into submission."[3] Rachel Carson said, "The 'control of nature' is a phrase conceived in arrogance, born of the Neanderthal age of biology and philosophy, when it was supposed that nature exists for the convenience of man."[4]

These are sad, pessimistic words that have increasingly come into our society in the last generation. However, there is one other voice, and since he was on the faculty at Southern Illinois University when he espoused it, let me leave you with that. This was the concept of Buckminster Fuller that he called *Spaceship Earth.*[5] The earth is a spaceship that a caring Father provided for children on that spaceship, with ample space, ample water, ample air, and ample fossil fuels in the hope and expectation that the children would grow up and learn to live within the systems of that spaceship before they would destroy themselves. No one knows how that experiment will come out, but it is obvious to all of us that we are now at a very critical stage, and what you are doing, what your concerns are today, are very much involved as to whether this spaceship will continue with people on it or whether it will be an empty hulk. Science, engineering, and medicine have helped in their way to create this problem, and it will take these same fields to find a solution and to make the spaceship flight safe and prosperous.

---

*From *Exploring New Ethics for Survival: The Voyage of the Space Ship Beagle,* edited by Garrett Hardin. Reprinted by permission of Viking Penguin, Inc.

REFERENCES

1. Hardin, Garrett. "The Tragedy of the Commons." In Hardin, Garrett (Ed.): *Exploring New Ethics for Survival: The Voyage of the Spaceship Beagle.* New York, Viking Press, 1972, p. 254, 255–256.
2. Schweitzer, Albert: In Carson, Rachel: *Silent Spring.* Boston, Houghton Mifflin Co., 1962.
3. White, E. B.: In Carson, Rachel: *Silent Spring.* Boston, Houghton Mifflin Co., 1962.
4. Carson, Rachel: *Silent Spring.* Boston, Houghton Mifflin Co., 1962, p. 297.
5. Fuller, Buchminster: *Operating Manual for Spaceship Earth.* Southern Illinois University Press, Carbondale, Illinois, 1969.

ACKNOWLEDGEMENTS

The Organizing Committee of the Decatur/Springfield Section of the American Chemical Society wishes to express their gratefulness to:

1. *American Chemical Society, Washington D.C.*
2. *A. H. Staley Manufacturing Co., Decatur, Ill.*
3. *ToxiGenics, Decatur, Ill.*

for their financial support of this symposium.

CONTENTS

ENVIRONMENTAL TOXICOLOGY

Chapter 1

INTRODUCTION TO THE
PRINCIPLES OF TOXICOLOGY

JAMES B. TERRILL

Each scientific discipline views toxicology within its own framework. An analytical chemist is concerned with detection and quantitative measurement of toxicants in air, soil, and water samples. On the other hand, a pharmacologist is concerned primarily with the biological response to various dosages of the toxicant. So, let us begin our introductory session with a review of terms and go over some basic examples. Historically, toxicology was the science of poisons. Toxicity is defined as the capacity of a substance to produce injury. The scope of modern toxicology has been expanded to include the study of the nature of adverse responses. As modern toxicologists, we have multicomponent relationships to develop and interpret. This is shown in Table 1–I.

First, there is the chemical or physical agent. We must be able to chemically identify it and determine its purity. We must verify that no significant decomposition of the test substance took place in the carrier or vehicle used to introduce it into the test system. This laboratory analysis is analogous to the identification and measurement of chemicals in our environment. Second, an appropriate biological system or species must be selected for testing. In mammalian toxicology, a rodent (rat or mouse) has been historically used in consideration of cost, ease of care, availability, and reasonable predictiveness for humans. Third, the selection of the route of administration and dose regimen must be made. The major routes by which toxic agents gain incidental entry into the body are through the gastrointestinal tract (ingestion), the lungs (inhalation), and the skin (topical). Also, therapeutic drugs that are potentially toxic can be administered subcutaneously, intra-

3

Table 1–I

MODERN TOXICOLOGICAL STUDY

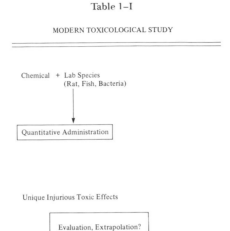

muscularly, and intravenously by injection.

The intravenous and inhalation routes are the fastest ways to get a material into the body. The selection of the route of administration of a test material should be based on the anticipated actual exposure. The dose regime that is the daily schedule for administration of the test substance should parallel the anticipated use. A single dose is used to determine the potency as an accidental poison. Repeated doses are used to evaluate cumulative effects. For an industrial worker, exposure is more likely to be by inhalation and dermal contact. For the consumer, the oral route is the most likely route of exposure. Fourth, the injuries that result from exposure to the toxicant must be described and interpreted. Last, the results of this laboratory data must be scientifically extrapolated to man's environment. This must be done as a scientific process and be based on the factual information that is available.

Now, I would like to go from this overview to several specific examples that describe how mammalian toxicology studies are conducted. The simplest type of response or endpoint to observe is an all-or-nothing response, such as death. A single treatment in which death is the potential endpoint is generally known as an acute study. The chemical can be given at a single level to a group of animals; every animal in the group would get the same dose. If a more complete picture is desired, several groups of animals should be treated; each group would receive a different dose. Figure 1–1 shows the results obtained from this type of experiment. No deaths are observed in the groups receiving low doses. At the middle doses, part of the group died. At the high doses, all animals of the group died. These deaths can occur either during the exposure or within a postexposure observation period. The acute study shown here is likely to be the very first experiment that may be run on a new chemical. The cost is approximately $1,000.00 depending on route of administration and experimental design. Rats or mice are usually the test species.

It is important to understand the basic procedure for statistical treatment of dose-response data. Figure 1–2 shows that the sigmoid or S-shaped plot for response vs. dose can be made more nearly linear if the response is plotted vs. log of dose (or log exposure). This is simply an empirical data treatment procedure. Observe that the curve now appears rather linear between 16 percent and 84 percent response. There are several important terms that are

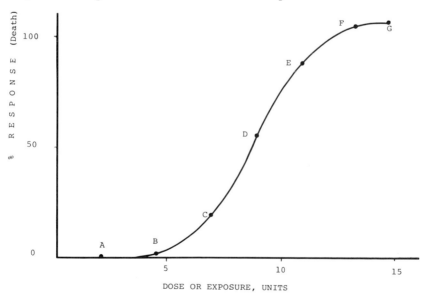

Figure 1–1. Dose–Response in Toxicity Testing.

used in describing the results of such an experiment. The first
term is the *middle point* of this plot, which is the mean lethal dose
or LD50. The value is calculated by regression analysis from the
experimental data. The second term is the *statistical confidence limits*
about the mean. A 95 percent confidence limits, which are two
sigma or two probit units, is the expression of choice. The next
important term is the *slope* of the dose-response relationship.

Experiments like this one show that there is a wide range of
toxicity for chemicals as shown in Table 1–II. These values were
obtained by oral, intravenous, subcutaneous, and intraperitoneal

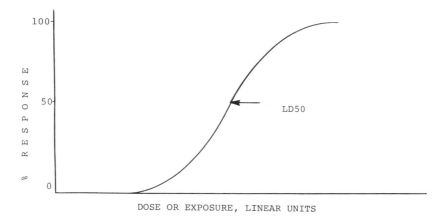

DOSE OR EXPOSURE, LINEAR UNITS

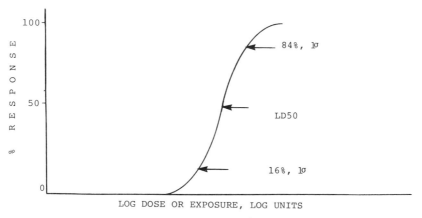

LOG DOSE OR EXPOSURE, LOG UNITS

Figure 1–2. Linear vs. Logrithmic Treatment of Data.

Table 1–II

APPROXIMATE ACUTE LD50S OF SELECTED CHEMICAL AGENTS

Agent	Species	Route	LD50 (mg/kg)
Ethyl Alcohol	Mouse	0	10,000
Sodium Chloride	Mouse	IP	4,000
Ferrous Sulfate	Rat	0	1,500
Morphine Sulfate	Rat	0	900
Sodium Phenobarbital	Rat	0	150
DDT	Rat	0	100
Picrotoxin	Rat	0	5
Strychnine Sulfate	Rat	SC	2
Nicotine	Rat	IV	1
d-Tubocurarine	Rat	IV	0.5
Dioxin (TCDD)	Guinea Pig	IV	0.001
Botulinus Toxin	Rat	IV	0.00001

(Taken from Loomis)

routes of administration in rodents and dramatically point out the necessity for the understanding of a chemical's toxic properties.

Figure 1–3 shows the significance of a difference in slope. Chemical A and B have the same LD50, but the lethal effects of Chemical A are apparent at much lower doses than Chemical B. Based on this data, one would have to be more conservative in setting exposure levels for Chemical A than Chemical B.

When I first described the acute experiment, I stated that the easiest response to study was an "all-or-nothing" response, such as death. The other type of response is termed *graded response*. This term is used mainly to describe physiological changes such as respiration or heart rate changes, blood pressure changes, etc. Similar statistical procedures may be used for treatment of this experimental data.

One last term that often appears in discussion of toxic effects is *threshold.* It is defined as a dose or exposure below which there is no apparent or, at least, not a measurable effect. Perhaps because it is supposed to be nonmeasurable, the existence of a threshold is a point of considerable scientific disagreement.

When a material has economic potential, additional toxicological information is usually required. The agent may be administered repeatedly or continuously. (Of course, the daily dose level is

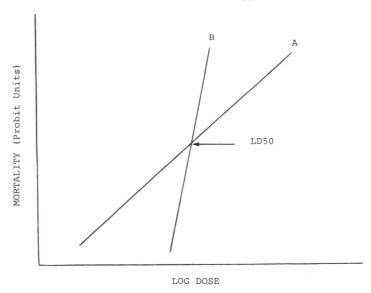

Figure 1–3. Importance of Slope in Toxicity Testing.

usually lower than in the acute study.) The examination for adverse effects is more extensive than in the acute study. This can involve microscopic examination of tissue and chemical examinations of blood and urine specimens. The cost is usually over ten thousand dollars just for a limited, one month study. A carcinogenic assessment can easily cost over a quarter of a million dollars. Table 1–III shows definitions for terms used in describing the repeated dose studies.

Table 1–III

TERMS FOR REPEAT DOSE STUDIES

Study Type	Parameters	Observations
Acute	Single Dose (2 weeks) 60 rats	Death, Severe Effects, Limited Obs.
Subacute	Multiple Dose, Multiple Groups 200 Rats, 1–3 Months	Subtle Health Effects Body Weight, Clinical Chem. Pathology
Chronic	Multiple Dose Multiple Groups 1000 Rats, 2 Yrs.	Carcinogenesis Pathology Detailed Obs.

In the repeated treatment study, the material may accumulate in the host if not eliminated. Materials such as lead, kepone, and cadmium that accumulate in tissue are of special interest to toxicologists.

The requirement for chronic and subacute testing is a two-edged sword. First, the expense and time required to carry out these tests means reduced and slower new product development and a subsequent higher cost to the consumer. On the other hand, the possibilities of unexpected toxicological discoveries during the use of the product will be reduced.

I would like to cover one last topic, Inhalation Toxicology. It is of special interest to me because I am an Inhalation Toxicologist. Inhalation experiments are a great analytical challenge, due to the emphasis placed upon documenting control of atmospheric levels for test material and the wide difference in physical properties and toxicity of test materials. In a basic inhalation experiment, the animal is placed into a large, sealed chamber that contains the test atmosphere. Food and water are generally removed during the exposure to avoid contamination of the diet by the test substance. The exposure schedule is usually six hours per weekly workday. The atmospheric concentration of the test substance in the chamber is monitored analytically two to six times per exposure. Also, the chamber temperature, air flow rate, relative humidity and nominal concentration of the test substance may be recorded.

Development of chambers that are easily constructed and designed such that the test material concentration is homogenous throughout the atmosphere has been developed over the last thirty years. The popular Rochester style chamber is shown in Figure 1–4. The conical top and bottom of these four-sided figures are its distinguishing features.

These remarks should help you realize that in order to understand the problems of modern toxicology a wide variety of skills must be used. Recently, the federal government has proposed new test protocols that demand a high level of technology in all toxicological research. Accurate identification and measurement of the test material in the atmosphere, the diet, or the water will insure the continued involvement of chemists in future toxicology experimentation.

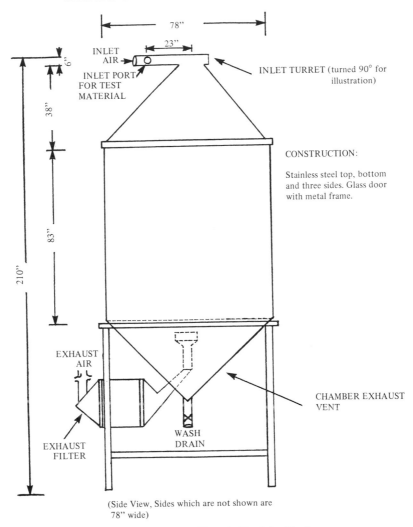

Figure 1–4. Inhalation Chambers for Chronic Toxicity Testing.

Chapter 2

METABOLISM AND DISPOSITION OF CHEMICALS IN RELATION TO TOXICITY

Satu M. Somani

Man and animal are exposed to foreign compounds, or nonnutrients, that enter the body intentionally or unintentionally. Intentionally, there are food additives and drugs that are taken as the occasion arises. Unintentionally, everyone is exposed to a number of chemicals, pestisides, etc., that find entry into the body through ingestion of food or drink, by inhalation, or by absorption through the skin. A large number of pesticides are consumed daily through food material.[1] Similarly, many chemicals are consumed through air and water in minute quantities.[2,3] These quantities are meager; however, one does not know whether these compounds and their metabolites play any role in relation to health effects in the whole span of life.

During the journey through the body, when a chemical compound is absorbed, it is distributed to various organs via systemic circulation and it reaches the site of action, i.e. the receptor site (Fig. 2–1). It is usually metabolized to a more polar compound to facilitate excretion from the body. During metabolism, a compound may form toxic metabolites or biologically intermediate reactive metabolites that could lead to adverse effects or degenerating health effects. A foreign compound that enters the body needs to be eliminated, and metabolism plays a major role in this elimination process. The compounds are finally excreted in urine, feces, bile, sweat, saliva, or milk.

Absorption of Foreign Compounds

When a man is exposed to foreign compounds, absorption may occur through the surface of the skin, by ingestion via the mouth

11

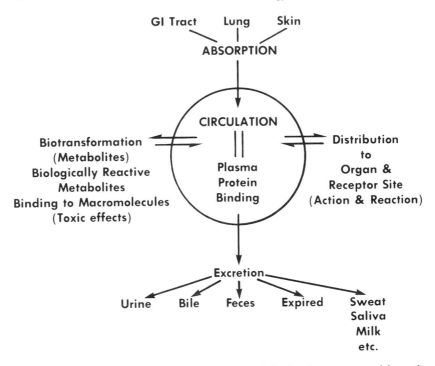

Figure 2–1. General scheme of the disposition of the foreign compound from the body.

into the GI tract, or by inhalation into the lungs. Until they are absorbed, there will not be any systemic effect. The absorption of a compound depends on its physico-chemical properties. In order to be absorbed, a compound must dissolve in the GI tract, cross the intestinal cell lining of the gut and get into the systemic circulation. Foreign organic compounds can be divided into two groups: lipophilic and hydrophilic. Soluble lipophilic compounds can easily cross cell membranes. Cell membranes consist of a bi-layer of lipoprotein molecules that allow the foreign compounds to diffuse through and pass into the plasma and tissues. Hydrophilic compounds such as quaternary ammonium compounds, neostigmine, pyridostigmine, etc., may dissolve in intestinal contents, still can not pass through the lipoprotein bi-layer of the cell membrane and thus are either poorly absorbed or not absorbed. Hence the more lipophilic the compound, the better it is absorbed from the GI tract, which is an important determinant of absorption.

Another physico-chemical property of all foreign organic compounds is that they are either an acid, base, or neutral and have a certain dissociation constant, pKa. A compound may exist in an ionized (I) and non-ionized form (IH) depending on the pH of the media. This is expressed by the Henderson-Hasselbach equation:

$$pH = pKa + Log\frac{I}{IH} \tag{1}$$

If I and IH have equal concentrations, then pH = pKa. Any change in pH will change the ratio of ionized to un-ionized components. Only the un-ionized form is readily absorbed through the cell membranes, and it crosses into the plasma and the tissues. The ionization of any foreign compound at any pH can be determined using the pKa of the compound.

Organic compounds are transported across biological membranes by four mechanisms: diffusion, filtration, active transport, and pinocytosis. Most foreign compounds are transported by the process of diffusion.

Distribution

Once a foreign compound is absorbed through the GI tract, lung, or skin, it enters the systemic circulation. The compound may either bind with plasma proteins or be dissolved in the blood. The most important contribution to binding of almost all foreign compounds is due to the albumin fraction that constitutes approximately 50 percent of the total plasma proteins. The other fractions of plasma proteins such as ceruloplasmin and transferrin bind copper and iron, respectively; and a and β-lipoproteins bind vitamins A, K, D, and E; cholesterol and steroid hormones. Globulins specifically interact with antigens. Thus, plasma proteins play an essential role in the transport of the ions and foreign compounds in the body.

The molecular binding of an organic molecule to albumin is totally nonspecific. The binding of the compound to albumin may be due to Van der Waal's forces, hydrogen bonding, or weak ionic interaction. It is very rare that covalent binding is observed. The binding of the compounds to the albumin molecule mainly depends upon the molecular structure of the compound and the binding is reversible. The foreign compound binds with a certain number of binding sites on each molecule of albumin, and each site has a different affinity for that compound. Only the free form of any compound is therapeutically or toxicologically active.

The binding of foreign compound to plasma proteins may affect (1) its concentrations in tissue fluid; (2) its therapeutic activity; (3) its toxicity; (4) its elimination through metabolic processes; and finally (5) its excretion in urine. The nonspecific binding characteristic of an organic molecule to an albumin molecule also leads to competitive processes for binding. A strongly-bound compound may displace a weaker-bound compound, thereby increasing the free concentration of the latter, which in turn is excessively available for its efficacy and receptor-compound interaction. In some cases, this displacement of a compound from albumin can lead to severe toxic reaction. It appears that acidic compounds bind more strongly to albumin molecules than basic compounds.

The affinity of compounds for certain organs or tissues varies. Compounds that are transported to different organs via blood may be in a bound or unbound form. The blood flow to different organs per unit time differs considerably.[4] The organs with the highest blood flow, such as heart, lung, kidney, and brain, will receive the highest amount of the compound, however, these organs have a very small capacity compared to fat and muscle, which have a large capacity but a very low blood flow. As an example of tissue distribution, Table 2–I shows the secobarbital concentrations in various tissues of rabbit at two different dose levels. The upper figure represents the 15 mg dose and the lower figure represents the 30 mg dose.[5] A better correlation between blood levels and highly perfused tissues such as liver and kidney was seen in contrast to fat and muscle. The secobarbital stored in the muscle eventually became a significant reservoir because of the large mass of muscle in the body. Certain compounds like DDT have a higher affinity for fatty tissue; therefore it accumulates in fat. Quinacrine, an antimalarial drug, binds to nucleic acids. Although a compound may accumulate in a tissue or organ, it may not exhibit any therapeutic action or toxic effect on that organ or tissue, but simply functions as a storage reservoir. As the concentration of a compound lowers in the other organs and systemic circulation, the accumulating organ releases the compound, keeping the proper equilibration in the blood stream.

The process of accumulation in organs or tissues involves an

Table 2-1

Concentrations of secobarbital in rabbit after intravenous administration of 15 and 30 mg/kg doses.
In each tissue, upper figures represent 15 mg dose and lower figures 30 mg dose. Concentration ($\mu g/gm$ of tissue or $\mu g/ml$ of blood) and Standard Error *

Time (mins.)	7.5	15	30	45	60	120
Blood	16.5 ± 1.6 32.0 ± 2.4	14.0 ± 1.8 25.5 ± 2.1	11.4 ± 0.2 18.4 ± 3.1	7.0 ± 0.9 11.6 ± 0.7	7.0 ± 0.9 14.3 ± 1.1	3.9 ± 0.8 6.0 ± 0.5
Liver	73.7 ± 6.3 109.0 ± 21.1	66.0 ± 6.1 83.7 ± 3.1	44.8 ± 6.8 67.3 ± 11.6	30.6 ± 7.6 38.7 ± 7.6	31.9 ± 4.3 44.7 ± 3.3	23.0 ± 5.2 21.7 ± 2.3
Kidney	26.7 ± 1.8 54.1 ± 5.7	23.0 ± 18.0 35.7 ± 2.7	21.6 ± 1.2 30.5 ± 4.4	10.5 ± 1.7 17.4 ± 1.1	15.5 ± 2.6 18.8 ± 1.1	6.7 ± 1.5 11.9 ± 1.9
Lung	17.6 ± 2.8 —	18.1 ± 1.3 —	12.8 ± 2.0 —	5.1 ± 2.4 —	14.2 ± 0.4 —	5.9 ± 0.8 —
Brain	18.0 ± 0.9 31.7 ± 4.0	22.8 ± 4.6 32.4 ± 1.9	12.0 ± 1.2 25.3 ± 5.3	10.8 ± 2.5 16.1 ± 2.6	9.2 ± 1.9 16.3 ± 1.9	8.9 ± 1.2 7.4 ± 0.4
Muscle	6.0 ± 0.5 14.4 ± 4.4	9.2 ± 2.1 18.2 ± 5.8	7.9 ± 2.0 11.9 ± 1.3	3.4 ± 0.4 8.9 ± 0.1	4.4 ± 1.2 14.2 ± 5.0	4.8 ± 2.6 4.5 ± 0.8
Fat	19.2 ± 10.0 13.1 ± 5.2	6.8 ± 3.8 9.2 ± 0.8	4.4 ± 3.5 31.0 ± 11.9	11.4 ± 7.8 26.7 ± 5.8	13.4 ± 4.5 34.8 ± 3.8	6.9 ± 7.1 17.7 ± 3.8

*Adapted from S. M. Somani, R. M. McDonald, and D. P. Schumacher: Pharmacokinetics of Secobarbital in Rabbit. Archives of Internationale Pharmacodynamic Therapy, 215:301-317, 1975.

active process by which an organ absorbs the compound or the compound binds to the proteins of that organ. Many compounds have specific affinity for certain organs, e.g. liver and kidney.

Reyes et al.[6] have successfully isolated the two hepatic cytoplasmic protein fractions designated as *y* and *z* that appear to play a role in the hepatic uptake of organic anions and in the selective transfer of the organic anions from plasma into the liver. These factors are also involved in the binding of certain dyes, chemicals, and carcinogens and their metabolites. This binding occurs in liver homogenates *in vitro* as well as *in vivo*. The *y* protein is exclusively present in liver and is induced by the administration of phenobarbital or other chemicals to rats. This induction of *y* contributes to the enhancement of hepatic uptake and metabolism of various anionic compounds.

Somani and Anderson[7] have studied the sequestration of a quaternary ammonium compound, neostigmine, an anticholinesterase inhibitor, by the liver. When this compound was added to perfusate in the isolated rat liver perfusion system, 50 to 70 percent of the neostigmine was sequestered in the liver. The mechanism by which this cation gets sequestered in the liver is not clear. Whether it involves the same *y* proteins, or different proteins, needs to be investigated.

Pharmacokinetics

Pharmacokinetics is the study of the time course of foreign compounds and their metabolites with respect to absorption, distribution, metabolism and elimination processes and of the mathematical relationships which can be used in models for interpreting tissue levels observed in biological systems.

The most simple model is one compartment model in which the foreign compound is assumed to be distributed instantaneously and uninformly throughout the system (Fig. 2–2). Elimination from the system is proportional to the concentration of foreign substance in the system. Equation 2 represents a one compartment model after intravenous bolus administration.

$$C = C_\rho \, e^{-Kt} \tag{2}$$

C is the concentration at any time t, Co is the concentration at time zero and K is the elimination rate constant. A semilogarithmic

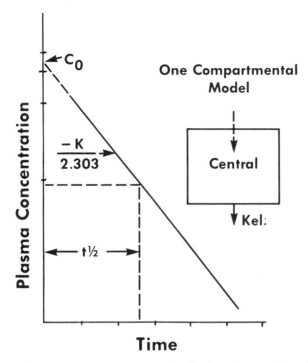

Figure 2–2. The plasma concentration vs. time is plotted on semilogarithic graph. Monoexponential decline or elimination is shown using one compartment model.

plot of C versus time (Fig. 2–2) yields a straight line with ordinate intercept Co and slope $-K$. The elimination rate (K) is a summation of both renal (Ke) and metabolism (Km) rates.

A good number of foreign compounds are eliminated by first-order kinetics. The time required for elimination to half its original is known as half-life ($t_{1/2}$). The relation of t to K is given by equation 3.

$$t_{1/2} = \frac{0.693}{K} \tag{3}$$

The half-life has more physical significance than K, in that the percent remaining in the body as per unit time can be calculated easily. However, when a foreign compound is administered to an animal, its monoexponential decline or elimination is rarely seen. Instead, the foreign compound usually exhibits biexponential decline (Fig. 2–3). The first rapid decline is called the distributive phase (a), and the slow decline is the elimination phase (β). This

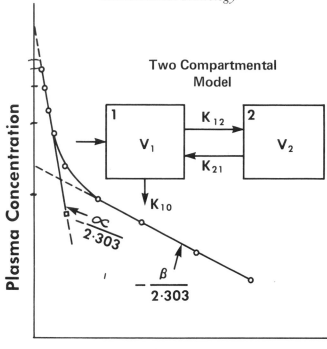

Time

Figure 2–3. The plasma concentration vs. time is plotted on semilogarithic graph. Biexponential decline or elimination of a foreign compound is shown using one compartment model.

bi-exponential elimination represents the two compartment model (Fig. 2–3).

The apparent volume of distribution (Vd) of a chemical is proportionality between the amount of the chemical and its plasma concentration. The ordinate intercept of semilogarithmic concentration versus time plot is used to estimate the volume of distribution when the intravenous bolus dose "D" is known.

$$Vd = \frac{D}{C_o} \qquad (4)$$

The total amount of foreign compound in the body at a given time is calculated by multiplying Vd with C of a foreign compound at that time.

Another useful term in pharmacokinetics is *clearance* (Cl), which has the dimension of volume per unit time. It is a product of the Vd and its corresponding elimination rate constant, i.e. $Cl_r = Vd \times Ke.$

Metabolism of Foreign Compounds

If there were no metabolism of foreign compounds taking place, the compounds are retained in the body for a much longer time, leading to severe toxicity. When a compound is metabolized in the body, the metabolic products are usually more polar or more ionized than the parent compound. These more ionized and more polar compounds are less able to bind to plasma and tissue proteins, less likely to be stored in the fat, and less able to penetrate cell membranes. These are readily eliminated from the body by the kidney or biliary system. Most of the foreign compounds are inactivated by metabolism, but activation and change of activity may also occur (e.g. parathion, an insecticide, is converted to paraoxon, an extremely toxic compound). The metabolism of foreign compounds may produce toxic metabolites that are responsible for adverse or toxic effects.

MICROSOMAL AND NONMICROSOMAL ENZYMES: The endoplasmic reticulum (ER) is a lipoprotein tubular network present in the cytoplasm. Microsomes are artifacts that are produced by the breakdown of ER. ER is of two types: (1) Rough Endoplasmic Reticulum (RER) containing ribosomes and (2) Smooth Endoplasmic Reticulum (SER) containing the highest level of enzymatic activity. Enzymes present in the endoplasmic reticulum or in microsomes are called microsomal enzymes. These enzymes metabolize all lipid soluble foreign compounds forming products that are less lipid soluble, but polar compounds may also be metabolized by these enzymes. These "mixed-function oxidases" of the microsomal enzyme system are also involved in the formation and degradation of steroid hormones, prostaglandins, synthesis of bile acids and cholesterol, and the oxidation of fatty acids.

Enzymes located at other sites of the cell are called nonmicrosomal enzymes. There are many oxidases and dehydrogenases present in the mitochondrial and soluble fractions of tissue homogenates, and many other enzymes such as esterases are present in the blood. There are some metabolic transformations of foreign compounds for which the enzyme and enzyme locations are not yet known.

TWO PHASE PROCESS METABOLISM OF FOREIGN COMPOUNDS: Organic chemicals are metabolized according to the active chemical grouping that they contain. The initial result of metabolism is either activation or inactivation, but eventually all metabolized compounds are inactivated and changed to more easily excretable forms.

The metabolism of an organic compound occurs in two phases as shown in Fig. 2–4. The first phase reaction includes oxidation, reduction, and hydrolysis. The phase II reactions are referred to as conjugations. During the phase I reaction, a compound may acquire –OH, –NH_2, –COOH, or –SH, through which it undergoes the synthetic phase II reactions. If the compound possesses any of these reactive groupings, it can undergo phase II reactions directly, without preparatory phase I change. Some of the compounds may be metabolized almost entirely by phase I reactions since the products (because of their particular chemical or physical properties) do not undergo conjugation. These metabolic reactions are subclassified and are shown in Table 2–II. Any of these metabolic biotransformations can form toxic metabolites, however, epoxidation reactions are considered to be the predominant producers of mutagens and carcinogens. The epoxides are electrophiles that could react with nucleophilic tissue constituents such as DNA, RNA, and protein and change the cellular macromolecules. However, epoxide hydrolases inactivate the epoxides to hydroxides and this enzyme is the rate limiting step in the conversion of toxic metabolites to a nontoxic form in this metabolic scene. The metabolic transformation of a foreign compound leads to the excretion of the products of oxidation, reduction and hydrolysis, and their conjugates. Original compounds may also be excreted in the urine. The proportion in which these three types of compounds are formed and excreted depends on several factors such as: route of administration, the dose, the rate of absorption, the chemical nature of the compound, plasma protein binding, age, species, strain, sex, diet and nutrition, circadian rhythms, and other environmental chemicals that may induce or inhibit the microsomal enzyme system.

PHASE II CONJUGATION REACTIONS: Conjugations are biosynthesis reactions in which foreign compounds or their metabolites combine with endogenous substrates to form conjugates. During phase I reactions, a foreign compound may acquire functional groups such as –OH, –NH_2, –COOH, and –SH. These reactive groups may combine with an endogenous compound that is frequently derived from a carbohydrate or an amino acid. The metabolites thus formed are referred to as conjugates and are shown in Table 2–III.

Table 2–II

METABOLIC BIOTRANSFORMATIONS OF FOREIGN COMPOUNDS

Microsomal Enzymes	*Nonmicrosomal Enzymes*
I. OXIDATION	I. OXIDATION
a. Hydroxylation of	a. Oxidation of Alcohols and Aldehydes
Aliphatic compounds	b. Deamination
Aromatic compounds	c. Aromatization of Alicyclic Compounds
Alicyclic Compounds	II. Reduction of Aldehydes and Ketones
b. Epoxidation	III. Hydrolysis
c. N-Hydroxylation of Amines	
d. N-Oxidation of Tertiary Amines	
e. S-Oxidation	
f. Dealkylation	
O-Dealkylation	
N-Dealkylation	
S-Dealkylation	
g. Deamination	
h. Desulphuration	
II. REDUCTION OF	
Nitro compounds	
Azo compounds	
Carbonyl compounds	
III. HYDROLYSIS	
Esters	
Amides	

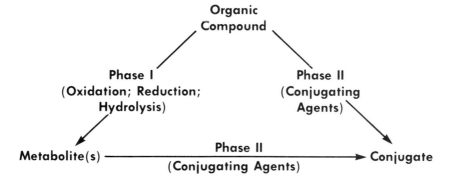

Figure 2–4. Schematic of the metabolism of foreign compounds.

If a compound contains any of these reactive groups, it may undergo phase II reactions without undergoing phase I reactions. These are water soluble and highly ionized at the pH of blood and tend to be readily excreted by the kidney. Glucuronide formation

Table 2–III

CONJUGATION REACTIONS

Functional group Containing organic Compound	Conjugate Formed
$-OH$, $-NH_2$, $-COOH$ and $-SH$	glucuronide
$-OH$, $-NH_2$	sulfate
$-OH$, $-NH_2$	methylation
$-NH_2$	acetylation
$-NH_2$	formylation
$-COOH$	glycine
$-Cl$, Hydrocarbon	Mercapturic acid

Table 2–IV

TYPES OF GLUCURONIDES

Ether glucuronide from— $-OH$ group
Ester glucuronide from— $-COOH$ group
N-glucuronide from— $-NH_2$ group
Thio-ether glucuronide from— $-SH$ group

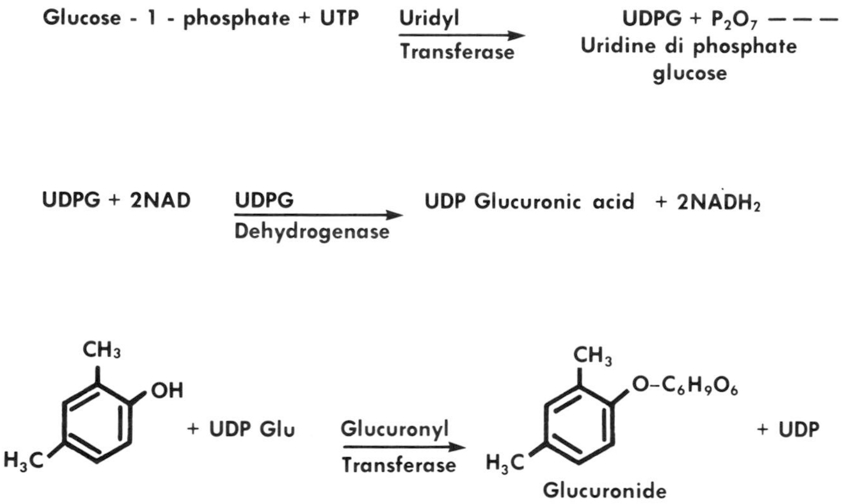
Glucose - 1 - phosphate + UTP
Uridyl
Transferase
UDPG + P₂O₇ — — —
Uridine di phosphate
glucose
UDPG + 2NAD
UDPG
Dehydrogenase
UDP Glucuronic acid + 2NADH₂
CH₃
OH
H₃C
+ UDP Glu
Glucuronyl
Transferase
CH₃
O-C₆H₉O₆
H₃C
Glucuronide
+ UDP

Figure 2–5. Mechanism of glucuronide formation.

is a predominant reaction that occurs in the liver and to a lesser extent in the kidney, gastrointestinal tract, and the skin. The formation of glucuronide of 2,4 DMP, for example, is a three step process (Fig. 2–5) that involves: (1) synthesis of uridine diphosphate glucose (UDPG) from glucose-1-phosphate by the enzyme uridyl transferase; (2) synthesis of uridine diphosphate a-D-glucosiduronic acid (UDPGLu) from UDPG by the enzyme UDPG dehydrogenase; and (3) transfer of glucuronyl moiety from UDPGlu to 2,4-dimethyl-phenol substrate. The formation of different types of glucuronides (Table 2–IV) depends on the functional group the aglycon contains.

The enzyme synthesizing UDP glucuronic acid are found in the soluble fraction of the tissues; but it appears that the glucuronyl transferases are located mainly in the microsomal fraction.

Mechanism of Metabolism and Toxicity

The majority of organic compounds considered foreign to the body undergo metabolic changes *in vivo*. These changes take place by a system of enzymes of low substrate specificity, known as *mixed oxygenases* or oxidases or microsomal hydroxylases. They are mainly present in the liver, but are also found, to some extent, in intestine, skin, kidney, and lung. This enzyme system has an absolute requirement for NADPH and molecular oxygen. The rate at which various compounds are metabolized by this enzyme system varies widely. The activity of a foreign compound in optimal doses is thus dependent on the rate of metabolism and on the relative extents of the different metabolic pathways.

The mechanism of these enzyme systems involves an electron

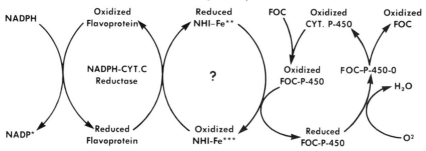

Electron transfer reactions in the oxidation of Foreign Organic Compound (FOC) and microsomal enzyme system. NHI=Non heme iron.

Figure 2–6. Electron transfer reactions in the oxidation of Foreign Organic Compound (FOC) and microsomal enzyme system. NHI = Non heme iron.

transport chain as shown in Figure 2–6.[8,9] The rate limiting step in this overall reaction is a heme-containing protein called cytochrome P–450. In the reduced form, this heme protein is capable of binding to carbon monoxide to yield a pigment with a characteristic absorption peak at 450 mμ.It has also been called a *co-binding pigment.*

Foreign compounds react with the oxidized form of Cyt. P–450. The Cyt. P–450 substrate complex is then reduced by a flavoprotein and NADPH cytochrome c-reductase possibly through an intermediate electron carrier, a nonheme iron containing protein, "Fe-Protein". The reduced Cyt. P–450 substrate complex then rapidly reacts with atmospheric oxygen and breaks down to form the oxidized compound, oxidized Cyt. P–450. Thus, the overall reaction involves the consumption of one molecule of compound with one atom of oxygen bound to the compound and the other oxygen atom appearing in water. This Cyt. P–450 is also involved in the reduction reactions.

Liver microsomal enzymes are induced by various agents. Pretreatment of animals with different inducers suggests that different forms of Cyt. P–450 exist in liver microsomes and other tissues. Multiple forms of Cyt. P–450 were also observed in the untreated animals. It has also been shown that the liver microsomes of the same animal contain multiple forms of Cyt. P–450. It appears that these cytochromes have different substrate specificities or overlapping specificities, and they play an important role in regulating the balance between activation and inactivation of an administered foreign compound.[10]

The two major forms of this cytochrome are Cyt. P–450 and Cyt. P–448, which have been differentiated on the basis of their inducible characteristics, enzyme activity and stability. Cyt. P–450 is mainly confined to hepatic tissues and Cyt. P–448 to extrahepatic tissues. The various forms of the Cyt. P–450, their localization, and proportionate concentration in various tissues, have an impact on the metabolism of foreign compounds and subsequently in the production of toxic metabolites. It appears that Cyt. P–448 plays a greater role in the formation of biologically reactive intermediates, mutagens, and carcinogens than Cyt. P–450.

Elimination of Foreign Compounds

Foreign compounds are eliminated from the body either by metabolism or by excretion in urine, bile, feces, saliva, or sweat.

The kidney is a very efficient organ for excretion of foreign compounds. A lipophilic or hydrophilic compound is filtered at the glomerulus. Compounds bound to plasma proteins and compounds with molecular weight of more than 60,000 daltons are not filtered at the glomerulus, because the capillary pores are only about 40 Å. The glomerular filtration rate and urine flow rate in normal man are about 100 ml and 1 ml per min, respectively. The ionized form of polar compounds will be excreted more readily than the un-ionized form as well as lipid soluble compounds. The latter compounds will be reabsorbed back into the peritubular capillary blood vessels and thus back into the circulation. The basic compounds will remain in the ionized form in acidic urine and the acidic compounds will be in the ionized form in basic urine and thus they will be excreted more rapidly. The advantage of this phenomenon could be taken to excrete the maximum amounts of toxic compounds from the body by making the urine acidic or basic for greater ionization of the compound, depending on its pKa. The converse will be true, however, for the reabsorption of the nonionized form by the tubule. A low clearance of a compound through the kidney is indicative of its longer half-life.

EXCRETION IN THE BILE: Foreign compounds are excreted in the bile. The liver secretes about 0.5 to 1 liter of bile in twenty-four hours. As a general rule, the compounds having molecular weight greater than 300 are excreted primarily in the bile. Glucuronides or other conjugates formed in the liver increase the molecular weight of the compounds or their metabolites. These could be excreted through the bile, which in turn passes into the duodenum via the bile duct. These compounds are then excreted in the feces or reabsorbed through the intestine. The glucuronide may be cleaved to its aglycon by the β-glucuronidase enzyme of the gut bacteria. This aglycon is reabsorbed and gets back into systemic circulation, thus establishing the enterohepatic recirculation of foreign compounds or their metabolites. Certain enzyme inducers increase the biliary excretion of foreign compounds. This method could be of aid in getting rid of the toxicants from the body.

ELIMINATION AND RECIRCULATION THROUGH SALIVARY SECRETION: A large number of drugs and foreign compounds are present in saliva, and their salivary concentrations are a reliable index of the free faction in plasma.[11,12]

We have carried out the determination of caffeine and theophylline in 239 simultaneously drawn samples of serum and saliva from human neonates. These drugs were used for the treatment of apnea of prematurity. We have found the close relationship between serum and saliva concentrations of these methylxanthines in neonates.[13]

Ben-Aryeh and Gutman[14] have described human saliva samples as an excellent specimen for monitoring the environmental chemicals to which they are exposed. The secretion of saliva is dependent on a number of factors such as age, disease, exposure to drugs and chemicals, etc.[15]

The secretion of saliva ranges in neonates from 0.01 to 0.1 ml/min, in infants from 0.04 to 0.4 ml/min as shown by Prader et al.[16] and in adults from 0.35 to 0.38 ml/min as suggested by Schneyer.[17] It appears that infants and neonates secrete much more saliva than adults on a body weight basis. Therefore, the salivary route of excretion of drugs may be more important in the pediatric population than in adults. As shown in Figure 2–7, saliva is swallowed and compounds present in saliva are reabsorbed from gastrointestinal tract and reenter the circulation. This recirculation of compounds through salivary absortion in the gut may prove to be an important pathway. However, this hypothesis (Fig. 2–7) of excretion and reabsorption has not yet been experimentally confirmed. Saliva is an easy and readily available sample obtained without discomfort to man. This is an excellent alternative to blood sampling for monitoring of the drug or foreign compound concentrations of free fraction in plasma. This unbound form (free fraction) of the compound is a pharmacologically and toxicologically active component,[18] whereas the bound compound is the reserve that helps to maintain the steady state during the processes of absorption, distribution, metabolism, and excretion.

SUMMARY: Human beings are continually exposed to environmental pollutants. They find their entry into the body through the GI tract, the lung, and the skin. Pollutants are distributed to various organs, and some chemicals localize in certain organs. These pollutants are metabolized by a microsomal enzyme system and are converted to more polar forms so as to be excreted. It is ironic that the enzymes that are envolved in detoxifying the chemical from the body are also involved in the formation of toxic compounds, mutagens, and carcinogens.

Elimination and Recirculation Through Salivary Secretion

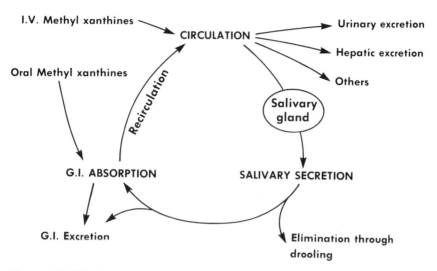

Figure 2–7. Elimination and Recirculation Through Salivary Secretion.

References

1. Duggan, R. E.: Pesticide residues in foods. In Kraybill, H. F.: Biological Effects of Pesticides in Mammalian Systems. *New York Academy of Science, 160·1:173–182, 1969.*

2. Phalen, R. F., Reischl, P., Freder, E. J., and Cavender, F. L.: Response of the respiratory tract to inhaled pollutants. In Willeke, Klans (Ed.): *Generation of Aerosols.* Ann Arbor, MI, Ann Arbor Science Publishers, Inc., 1980, pp. 125–139.

3. Somani, S. M., Teece, R. G., and Schaeffer, D. J.: Identification of cocarcinogens and promoters in industrial discharges into and in the Illinois River. *J Toxicol Environmental Health,* 6:315–331, 1980.

4. Levine, R.: *Pharmacology Drug Actions and Reactions.* Boston, Little Brown and Co. Inc., 1978, pp. 104.

5. Somani, S. M., McDonald, R.M., and Schumacher, D.P.: Pharmacokinetics of secobarbital in rabbit. *Archiv Internationale Pharmacodynamic Therap,* 215:301–317, 1975.

6. Reyes, H., Levi, A. J., Gatmaitan, Z., and Arias, I. M.: Studies of y and z, two hepatic cytoplasmic organic anion-binding proteins: Effects of drugs, chemicals, hormones and cholestasis. *J Clin Inv,* 50:2242, 1971.

7. Somani, S. M., and Anderson, J. M.: Sequestration of neostigmine and metabolites by perfused rat liver. *Drug Metabolism and Disposition,* 3:275–282, 1975.

8. Curry, S. M.: *Drug Disposition and Pharmacokinetics.* Philadelphia, Lippencott, 1975, pp. 53–55.

9. Goldstein, A., Aronow, L., and Kalman, S.: *Principles of Drug Action: The Basis of Pharmacology,* 2nd ed. New York, John Wiley and Sons, Inc. 1974, pp. 242–245.

10. Lu, A. Y. H. and West, S. B.: Multiplicity of mammalian microsomal cytochromes P–450. *Pharmacological Reviews, 31:* 277–295, 1980.

11. Bender, I. B., Pressman, R. S., and Tashman, S. G.: Studies on excretion of antibiotics in human saliva. *J Am Dent Assoc, 46:* 164–170, 1953.

12. Cook, C. E., Amerson, E., Poole, W. K., Lesser, P., and O'Tuama, L.: Phenytoin and phenobarbital concentrations in saliva and plasma measured by radioimmunoassay. *Clin Pharm Therap, 18:* 742–747, 1975.

13. Somani, S. M. and Khanna, N. N.: Correlation of serum, CSF and saliva concentrations of methylxanthines in neonates. In Soyaka, C. F. and Redmond, G. P. (Eds.): Proceedings of the Symposium on *Determinants of Drug Metabolism in Immature Human.* New York, Raven Press, in press.

14. Ben-Aryeh, H. and Gutman, D.: Saliva for biological monitoring. In Berlin, A., Wolff, A. H., and Hasegawa, Y. (Eds.): *The Use of Biological Specimen for the Assessment of Human Exposure to Environmental Pollutants.* Hague, Martinus-Nijhoff, 1979, pp. 65–69.

15. Mason, D. K. and Chisholm, D. M.: *Salivary Glands in Health and Disease.* Philadelphia, W. B. Saunders and Co., 1975, pp. 41–55.

16. Prader, A., Gautier, E., Gautler, R., and Naef, D.: The Na^+? and K^+? concentration in mixed saliva. *Helv Paediat Acta, 10:* 29–55, 1955.

17. Schneyer, L. H.: Source of resting total mixed saliva of man. *J Appl Physiol, 9:* 79–81, 1956.

18. Fingl, E. and Woodbury, D. M.: Plasma proteins and other extracellular reservoirs. In Goodman, I. S. and Gilman, A. (Eds.): *The Pharmacological Basis of Therapeutics,* 5th ed. New York, The MacMillan Company, 1975, p. 10.

Chapter 3

TARGET ORGAN TOXICITY

Drug-induced Changes in the Lung, Liver, and Kidney in Inhalation and Dietary Toxicity

Beverly Y. Cockrell and W. M. Busey

ABSTRACT

Light and electron microscopic changes in the respiratory tract following inhalation of sulfuric acid mist will be used as an example of pulmonary response to irritant gases and vapors, whereas aluminum chlorhydrate (ACH) aerosol inhalation will serve as prototype for particulate exposures. The pulmonary reaction is fairly characteristic for each with edema and hemorrhage being common following acid exposure and an end airway macrophagic reaction after ACH exposure.

An example of carcinogenicity, as the end result of inhalation toxicity, will be given by a discussion of induction of liver tumors following subchronic exposure to 2-nitropropane. Other examples of hepatic toxicities following dietary exposures will include drug-induced proliferations of smooth endoplasmic reticulum resulting in hepatocellular enlargement and increased liver weights and the production of hepatocellular myeloid bodies that regress following cessation of drug treatment.

A discussion of examples of drug-induced renal toxicities will include light and electron microscopic changes following dietary exposure to various chlorinated hydrocarbons and to toxic levels of various antibiotics.

29

Respiratory Tract Toxicities

Inhalation exposure to sulfuric acid mist became of interest because of exposure of industrial workers and because of its widespread distribution as an air pollutant.[1] Early experiments demonstrated that there was considerable variation in response among various laboratory animals with the guinea pig being very sensitive and the rat very resistant.

Experiments were initiated to study the deep lung irritation caused by sulfuric acid mist in guinea pigs. Detailed results have been reported elsewhere.[2-5] This report will summarize these findings. Guinea pigs exposed to high concentrations (30 or 100 mg/m^3) usually died from severe pulmonary edema, hemorrhage, and diffuse acute alveolitis. The pulmonary lesions indicated that sulfuric acid mist was a deep lung irritant, affecting alveoli and terminal bronchioles. At lower concentrations (10–20 mg/m^3) of sulfuric acid mist, guinea pigs developed a regional alveolitis around some, but not all, alveolar ducts. Sharp lines of demarcation could be seen between normal lung tissue and affected areas. The segmental distribution of alveolitis could be seen by light and scanning electron microscopy (SEM) (Figure 3–1A, B) and des-

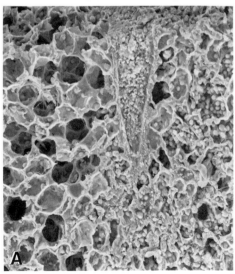

Figure 3–1. Sulfuric acid-induced segmental alveolitis. **A.** The affected part of the lung is to the right with edema and infiltration of blood cells. (SEM, reduced 30 percent from X250).

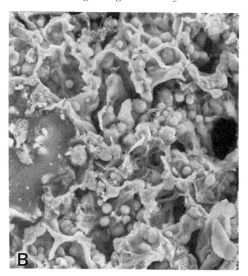

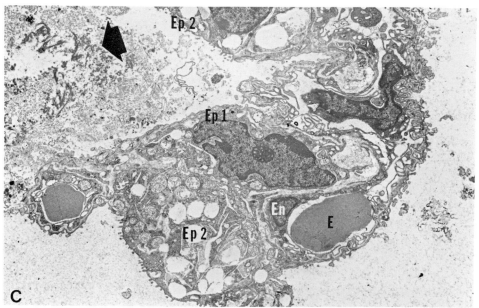

Figure 3–1. Sulfuric acid-induced segmental alveolitis. **B.** A higher magnification shows numerous blood cells in the alveoli. (Reduced 30 percent from X470). **C.** A transmission electron micrograph (TEM) shows the deposition of fibrin and proteinaceous material (arrow) near an end airway. Ep 1 = Type I pneumocyte; Ep 2 = Type II pneumocyte; En = endothelium; E = erythrocyte. (reduced 29 percent from X6,180).

Figures 1A and 1B reproduced by permission of the Journal of Toxicology and Environmental Health, Hemisphere Publishing Corporation, Washington, D.C.

quamation of cells lining the alveolar ducts with fibrin deposition by transmission electron microscopy (TEM) (Figure 3–1C).

When guinea pigs were exposed to 25 mg/m^3 sulfuric acid mist for two days for six hours per day, pulmonary lesions were acute and similarly characterized by edema and hemorrhage with distinct demarcations between altered and normal parenchyma.

Other experiments were designed to expose guinea pigs to sulfuric acid mist (10 mg/m^3), ozone (0.5 ppm), and their combination in order to evaluate possible synergistic effects of these pollutants from a six-month exposure.

Guinea pigs exposed to O_3 or the combination of O_3 plus H_2SO_4 mist for six months characteristically had lesions near the terminal bronchioles of the lungs. The epithelium was hypertrophied and hyperplastic and alveolar macrophages were present in alveoli around the terminal bronchioles. Occasionally there was minimal proliferation of type II cells. A slight loss of cilia was observed in the epithelium of the bronchi and tracheae of animals in these groups. Associated with the loss of cilia in the tracheae was a reduction of goblet cells and mild basal cell hyperplasia.

Guinea pigs exposed to 10 mg/m^3 H_2SO_4 mist alone had minimal proliferation of alveolar macrophages and mild tracheal changes such as loss of epithelial cilia.

The results of this investigation indicated that respiratory changes after a six month exposure to H_2SO_4 mist alone were minimal to negligible. When animals were exposed to both O_3 and H_2SO_4 mist, the latter did not appear to enhance the microscopic lesions caused by O_3 alone.

An example of the lung as a target organ for particulate inhalation exposure was provided by six-month, one-year, and two-year exposures of rats and guinea pigs to aluminum chlorhydrate. This chemical is a common component of aerosol antiperspirants and was used in these inhalation toxicity studies since preliminary work with a chemically related compound[6] indicated that pulmonary lesions resulted. The exposure was given six hours a day, five days a week. Following a six-month exposure[7], the lungs of animals exposed to either 2.5 or 25 mg/m^3 of ACH contained exposure related granulomatous reactions characterized by many large, foamy alveolar macrophages and mononuclear cells situated around terminal bronchioles. Reactions in the lungs of animals treated with the lowest dosage, 0.25 mg/m^3 ACH were minimal to negligible.

After one-year inhalation exposure, rats and guinea pigs exposed to 2.5 or 25 mg/m^3 ACH had granulomatous reactions around the end airways of the lung (Figure 3–2A & B). Macrophages containing ACH-related spicules were observed in the lungs (Figure 3–2C & D) and in the peribronchial lymph nodes (Figure 3–3A & B). Although there were exposure related clumps of macrophages around some of the end airways in the low dose (0.25 mg/m^3) exposure, neither mononuclear inflammatory cells nor changes in the walls of the terminal bronchioles or alveolar ducts accompanied these.

After a two-year exposure[8] to the high and intermediate dose, the reaction was more advanced, involving all of the end airways. Exposure related lesions were more severe in the rats than the guinea pigs with more fibrosis and alveolar proteinaceous debris. Inflammatory cells, also, appeared more commonly in the rats. ACH-related spicules were seen in the lung and peribronchial lymph nodes.

In the low dose (0.25 mg/m^3) exposure, there were exposure related aggregates of macrophages around many of the airways with no inflammatory cells. Type II cell hyperplasia was sometimes observed in the walls of terminal bronchioles or alveolar ducts in these areas resulting in a definitive multifocal, exposure related lesion. In these low dose animals, there were also exposure related aggregates of macrophages in the peribronchial lymph nodes.

Liver Toxicities

The liver can be the target organ in not only dietary but inhalation studies. When rats were exposed by inhalation to 207 ppm of 2-nitropropane, a solvent used in the production of plastics, rubber, and adhesives, hepatocellular toxicities developed. After a three-month exposure, hepatocellular hypertrophy, hyperplasia, and necrosis were seen. After six-months inhalation exposure to 207 ppm of 2-nitropropane, all rats had neoplastic nodules and hepatocellular carcinomas (Figures 3–4A, B, & C). These findings

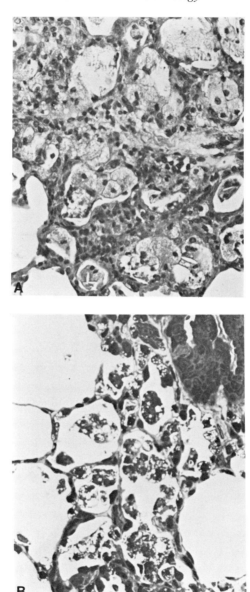

Figure 3–2. Aluminum chlorhydrate-induced macrophagic reaction round the end airways. **A.** Alveolar sacs and neighboring alveoli are filled with large, foamy alveolar macrophages and occasional cholesterol clefts. The alveolar walls are thickened by increased numbers of Type II cells. (H&E, reduced 40 percent from X400). **B.** The one (1) micron section of plastic embedded lung shows numerous cytoplasmic vacuoles in the macrophages. (Toluidine blue, reduced 40 percent from X400).

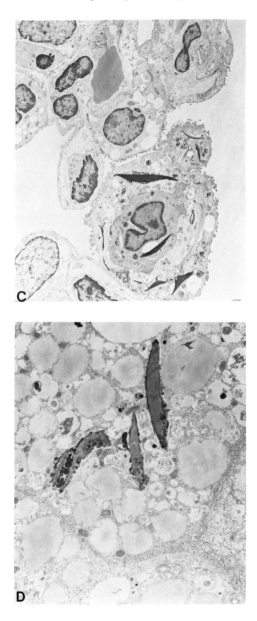

Figure 3–2. Aluminum chlorhydrate-induced macrophagic reaction round the end airways. **C.** The alveolar macrophages are not only vacuolated but contain electron-dense ACH-related spicules. (TEM, reduced 40 percent from X3,800). **D.** This micrograph shows the ACH-related spicules in the cytoplasm of a degenerating macrophage. (TEM, reduced 40 percent from X9,600).

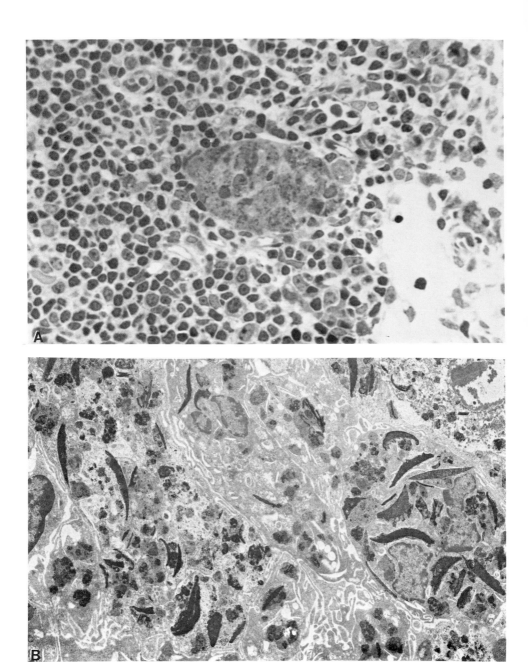

Figure 3–3. ACH-induced macrophagic reaction in the peribronchial lymph node.
A. By light microscopy, multiple foci of macrophages with cytoplasmic dense particles were present. (Toluidine blue, reduced 32 percent from X400). **B.** By TEM, the cytoplasmic particles are electron-dense ACH-related spicules similar to those seen in the lungs. (TEM, reduced 32 percent from X7,200).

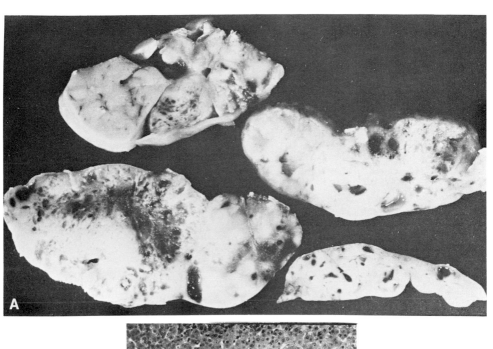

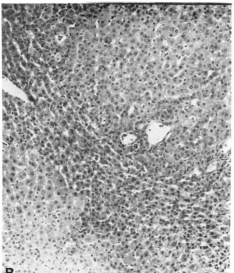

Figure 3–4. Hepatocellular toxicities induced by 2-nitropropane. **A.** The cut surface of the affected liver contains foci of hemorrhage and tumorous nodules. **B.** Several neoplastic nodules are seen compressing normal liver near the center (H&E, reduced 40 percent from X100).

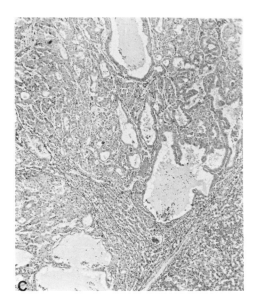

Figure 3–4. Hepatocellular toxicities induced by 2-nitropropane. C. This hepatocellular carcinoma has a trabecular pattern and multiple cysts. Normal liver appears at the lower right (H&E, reduced 40 percent from X400).

indicate that 2-nitropropane is a potent carcinogen in the rat with inhalation exposure resulting in carcinoma of the liver.[9]

Other than carcinogenicity, toxic changes commonly observed in the livers are fatty change, proliferations of smooth endoplasmic reticulum and the presence of cytoplasmic myeloid bodies. Accumulation of fat in the liver follows treatment with a wide variety of chemicals, and the reader is referred to an excellent review by Plaa.[10] Proliferation of smooth endoplasmic reticulum has become known as the morphological expression of drug-induced enzyme production in the liver. Well known examples of this are phenobarbital[11] and dieldren induced proliferations.[12] In addition, myeloid or myelinoid bodies have been produced in the liver by a wide variety of drugs, including triparanol, chloroquine, and erythromycin. The reader is referred to two excellent reviews.[13,11] In our laboratory, we have observed drug-induced myeloid bodies in both liver and kidney.

Renal Toxicities

Examples of drug-induced changes in the kidneys are refractile pigments seen in the lumens of some proximal convoluted tubules (Figure 3–5A) in rats treated with an arsenic used as a grain fungicide. By electron microscopy the "pigments" are electron-dense bodies which appear in lysosomes, in the brush border and the lumen of the renal proximal tubules (Figure 3–5B). Feeding a chlorinated hydrocarbon compound to rats resulted in crystalline-like structures in the epithelial cells of the proximal convoluted tubules (Figure 3–5C). Electron microscopy demonstrated that these drug-induced crystals filled much of the cytoplasm of the epithelial cells of the proximal tubules (Figure 3–5D) resulting in degeneration, necrosis and sloughing of these cells into the tubular lumens. These findings suggest that drug-induced metabolites may be present in the urine from treated animals.

Renal toxicities have also been associated with a wide variety of antibiotics, sulfas and other drugs.[14] Treatment of dogs with bleomycin resulted in focal atrophy of the epithelial cells of the proximal convoluted tubules. These atrophied cells contained very prominent Golgi apparati (Figure 3–6A & B), a finding also associated with gentamicin nephrotoxicity.[15] In areas of more severe damage, the tubules were markedly atrophied and necrotic with only fragments of brush border remaining (Figures 3–6C & D). The cytoplasm of the degenerating epithelial cells contained whorls of membrane resembling myeloid bodies. The latter have also been reported following treatment with gentamicin.[15] The basement membranes were thickened surrounding affected tubules.

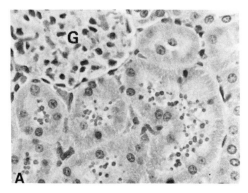

Figure 3–5. Drug-induced renal toxicities. A. Treatment of rats with an arsenical fungicide resulted in numerous spherical bodies in the proximal convoluted tubules. G=glomerulus (Toluidine blue, reduced 37% from X400).

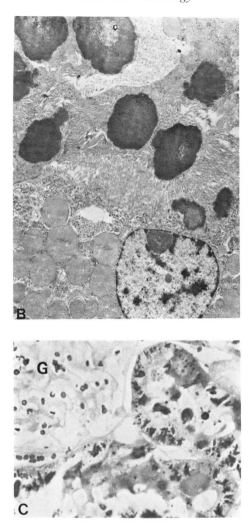

Figure 3–5. Drug-induced renal toxicities. **B.** By TEM, the spherical bodies are electron-dense and appear limited to the brush border (TEM, reduced 37% from X8,000). **C.** Treatment with a chlorinated hydrocarbon caused crystalline inclusions in the proximal tubular epithelium. G=glomerulus (Toluidine blue, reduced 37% from X400).

These thickened basement membranes were also seen in interstitial areas with no associated tubular epithelium suggesting that the membrane remains long after the necrotic epithelium has been phagocytized and removed.

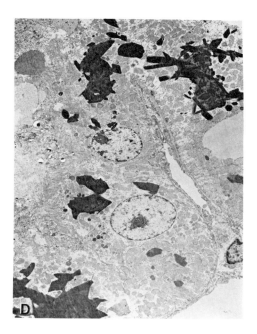

Figure 3–5. Drug-induced renal toxicities. **D.** By TEM, these crystalline inclusions filled much of the cytoplasm of these cells eventually resulting in their degeneration (TEM, reduced 37% from X3,200).

Photographs reproduced by permission of T. M. Scotti, M.D., U.S. Environmental Protection Agency, HERL, ETD, TEB, Research Triangle Park, North Carolina.

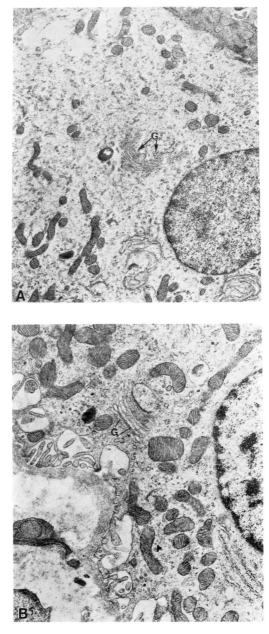

Figure 3–6. Antibiotic-induced renal tubular nephrosis. **A** and **B.** Prominent Golgi apparati (G) appear in affected tubular epithelium (TEM, reduced 36% from X12,100, and X17,000).

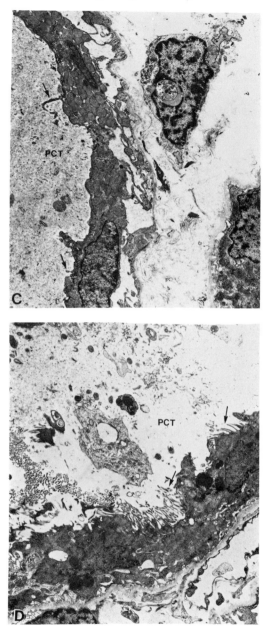

Figure 3–6. Antibiotic-induced renal tubular nephrosis. **C** and **D**. Degeneration and necrosis of the proximal convoluted tubules (PCT) are characterized by focal loss of the brush border (arrows) and compression and density of the epithelium (TEM, reduced 36% from X6,300, and X6,000).

REFERENCES

1. Natusch, D. F. S. and Wallace, J. R.: Urban aerosol toxicity: The influence of particle size. *Science, 186:*695–696, 1974.
2. Cavender, F. L., Williams, J. L., Steinhagen, W. H., and Woods, D.: Thermodynamics and toxicity of sulfuric acid mists. *J Toxicol Environ Health, 2:*1147–1159, 1977.
3. Cavender, F. L., Steinhagen, W. H., Ulrich, C. E., Busey, W. M., Cockrell, B. Y., Drew, R. T., Haseman, J. K., and Hogan, M. D.: Effects in rats and guinea pigs of short-term exposures to sulfuric acid mist, ozone, and their combination. *J Toxicol Environ Health, 3:*521–533, 1977.
4. Cockrell, B. Y., Busey, W. M., Cavender, F. L., Steinhagen, W. H., and Drew, R. T.: Light and electron microscopic pulmonary changes in rats and guinea pigs exposed to sulfuric acid mist. *Am Rev Respir Dis, 113:*91, 1976.
5. Cockrell, B. Y., Busey, W. M., and Cavender, F. L.: Respiratory tract lesions in guinea pigs exposed to sulfuric acid mist. *J Toxicol Environ Health, 4:*835–844, 1978.
6. Drew, R. T., Gupta, B. N., Bend, J. R., and Hook, G. E. R.: Inhalation studies with a glycol complex of aluminum-chloride-hydroxide. *Arch Environ Health, 28:*321–326, 1974.
7. Steinhagen, W. H., Cockrell, B. Y., and Cavender, F. L.: Six month inhalation exposures of rats and guinea pigs to aluminum chlorhydrate. *J Environ Path and Toxicol, 1:*267–277, 1978.
8. Busey, W. M., Cockrell, B. Y., and Cavender, F. L.: Morphologic changes following chronic inhalation of aluminum chlorhydrate in the rat and guinea pig. *Proceedings – 16th Annual Meeting,* Society of Toxicology, Toronto, Canada, March 27–30, 1977.
9. Busey, W. M., Ulrich, C. E., and Lewis, T. R.: Subchronic inhalation toxicity of 2-nitropropane in rats and rabbits. *Proceedings – 17th Annual Meeting,* Society of Toxicology, San Francisco, March 12–16, 1978.
10. Plaa, G. L.: Toxicology of the liver. In Doull, J., C. Klaasen and Amdur, M. O. (Eds.): *Toxicology,* 2nd ed. New York, Macmillan Publishing Co., 1980, pp. 206–231.
11. Ghadially, F. N.: *Ultrastructural Pathology of the Cell,* London, Butterworths, 1975, pp. 274 and 314.
12. Hutterer, F., Schaffuer, F. Klion, F. M., and Popper, H.: Hypertrophic hypoactive smooth endoplasmic reticulum: a sensitive indicator of hepatotoxicity exemplified by dieldrin. *Science, 161:*1017, 1968.
13. Hruban, A.; Slesers, A., and Hopkins, E.: Drug-induced and naturally occurring myeloid bodies. *Lab. Invest., 27:*62–70, 1972.
14. Kleinknecht, D., Kanfer, A., Morel-Maroger, L., and Mery, J., Ph.: Immunological mediated drug-induced acute renal failure. In Migone, L. (Ed.): *Contributions to Nephrology, Volume 10, Toxic Nephropathies.* New York, S. Karger, 1977, pp. 42–52.
15. Kosek, J. D., Mazze, R. I., and Cousins, M. J.: Nephrotoxicity of gentamicin. *Lab Invest, 30:*48–57, 1974.

Chapter 4

PHYSIOLOGICAL ASPECTS OF
HEAVY METAL TOXICITY

M. HEJTMANCIK, JR. AND B. J. WILLIAMS

Introduction

Heavy metals or their salts were once used extensively as therapeutic agents. Inorganic arsenic compounds were formerly used extensively in the treatment of cholera, malaria, syphilis, and certain nutritional diseases (pellagra), and intravenous injections of antimony compounds (tartar emetic) were used effectively against a number of tropical diseases such as filariasis, leishmaniasis, and schistosomiasis. Much information regarding the toxicity of metal compounds was derived from their therapeutic utilization, as continuous exposure produced cumulative effects that resulted in chronic poisoning with metabolic, nutritional, and neurological symptoms. Consequently, medical interest in heavy metals as therapeutic agents has decreased due to their frequent side effects and the advent of more efficacious and safer organic antibiotics and bacteriocidal agents. Although, a few metallic compounds of gold, lithium, and bismuth still exhibit valid therapeutic application for rheumatoid arthritis, manic depression, and x-ray diagnosis, respectively. Due to the steady accumulation of heavy metals into the environment, focus has shifted to the role of heavy metals as causative agents in the production of occupational or environmental-related diseases.

In atomic order, industrially based and wide-spread contaminants include beryllium, cadmium, antimony, mercury, and lead.[1] This chapter will focus on the potential adverse health effects of mercury, cadmium, and lead in particular due to the increased present-day environmental levels; although chronic exposure to other metals may occur in industrial workers and miners, it does not occur to the general public. Lead continues to be of interest because of potential central nervous system effects in children with greater than normal blood lead levels, and recent evidence that lead can produce metabolic and physiological effects at levels that are insufficient to produce the classical clinical symptoms.[2] It is not intended that these sections contain all that is known about the metals under consideration, but emphasis has been directed toward current interests and problems.

Essential Elements

Nine of the trace elements, which have been characterized as required for normal biological function, have been termed *essential*. Due to research in animal and human nutrition, essential elements are being discovered at the rate of two per decade.[1] These elements are present in the body in minute amounts and are utilized as enzymatic cofactors in the metabolism or manufacture of essential compounds (Table 4–I).[3] Man acquires adequate amounts of the essential elements in his diet, and there is usually no need for supplementation. These metals are under homeostatic control and there are specific mechanisms for their absorption in the intestine and excretion by the kidney. While this category encompasses elements clearly essential for normal biological functions, and deficiencies can result in disease, the accumulation of excess trace metals can produce distinct toxic effects.

Nonessential Heavy Metals

This category comprises heavy metals for which an essential role has not been determined, and which are toxic at low levels. Elements in this group include arsenic, antimony, mercury, lead, and cadmium. Unfortunately, some of these metals are by-products of modern industrialization and tend to accumulate in the environment increasing the risk of chronic human exposure to amounts of metals to which man has been little adapted in the past. Pollution by heavy metals is a more insidious problem than pollution by other organic substances, such as sulfur dioxide, that are degradable by natural processes.[1]

A few historic examples indicate that excessive heavy metal exposure can result in chronic human disease. A large zinc smelter

Table 4–I

FUNCTIONS OF TRACE ELEMENTS IN MAN*

Element	Function
Iron	Component of hemoglobin, myoglobin, catalase, and cytochromes. Essential for synthesis of Vitamin B.
Zinc	Enzyme cofactor required for trytophan synthesis and protein synthesis.
Copper	Catalyst for oxidation-reduction reactions, and required for synthesis of hemoglobin and iron-containing enzymes.
Manganese	Enzyme cofactor, promotes vitamin synthesis, and affects calcium metabolism.
Chromium	Involved in sugar and fat metabolism.
Cobalt	Constituent of Vitamin B_{12}, enzyme activator, promotes synthesis of iron-containing pyrroles.
Molybdenum	Cofactor for the metabolism of purines to uric acid.
Iodine	Required for synthesis of thyroxin.
Fluorine	Necessary for formation of strong bones and teeth, and for prevention of dental caries.

*Modified from table in N. M. Trieff: *Environment and Health.* Ann Arbor Science Publ. Inc., Ann Arbor, Mich., 1980, p. 370.

located on Toyama Bay, Japan, dumped its effluents into the water, which was used by farmers downstream to irrigate rice crops. Inhabitants that consumed the produce eventually developed severe joint pain, osteomalacia, deformities of the spine, and easily broken bones. This condition was called Itai-itai disease, and cadmium was identified as the causative factor.[1]

Cobalt was established as the etiological agent in a series of instances of severe cardiac failure in persons consuming large amounts of beer to which soluble cobalt salts were added to reduce foaming.[3]

An outbreak of arsenic poisoning occurred in Japan in 1955 as a result of infants consuming powdered milk contaminated with the metal.[4] The arsenic was introduced into the milk as a contaminant of a sodium phosphate stabilizer.

The conversion of a heavy metal pollutant in the ecosystem to a more toxic form and its subsequent concentration in food has also been described. Again in Japan, a factory manufacturing plastics dumped an inorganic mercury-spent catalyst into Minamata Bay from 1953–1960, not realizing that bacteria were converting the inorganic form into organic forms such as methyl mercury.[1] It was finally determined that the organomercurial compounds were being concentrated in marine animals that constituted the dietary staple of the local population, resulting in methyl mercury poisoning. A similar situation also occurred in Sweden, in which mercury poisoning was experienced by a population eating fish that had become contaminated with an organic mercury compound used as a pesticide that had washed into local waters.[5] While mass poisonings have resulted from high level heavy metal exposure, little is known regarding the effects of prolonged exposure to low concentrations of these metals.

Specific Organ Toxicity

A tentative classification of the target organ toxicity of several metals is shown in Table 4–II, which includes all of the effects that can result from moderate to severe industrial exposure, accidental poisoning, or chronic low level (environmental) exposure.[6] The metals that exhibit the greatest potential toxicity are those that tend to accumulate in the body, such as lead and cadmium. The use of nondegradable heavy metals in industry has increased the possibility of nonoccupational exposure, and this problem will be discussed in a subsequent section. While the adverse effects associated with acute exposure to most heavy metals have been identified, the biochemical or physiological mechanisms of toxicity remain elusive.

High Level Exposure

This section is devoted to those effects of heavy metals that are indicative of chronic and acute high level intoxication. The effects of arsenic, antimony, mercury, lead, and cadmium will be discussed in order to formulate some general concepts regarding heavy metal toxicity. Other metals capable of producing rather selective organ effects will also be mentioned.

ARSENIC. The toxicity of a particular heavy metal is often related to how fast it is cleared from the body and to what extent it accumulates in tissues. The various arsenic compounds exhibit a

Table 4-II

TARGET ORGANS OF METALS

Metal	Respiratory Tract	CNS	Cardiovas. System	Liver	Blood	Kidney	Bone
Antimony	+		+	+			
Arsenic	+	+		+		+ + +	+
Barium	+		+				
Beryllium	+	+ +					
Bismuth	+		+	+			
Cadmium			+			+ + +	+
Chromium	+	+ + +	+	+			
Cobalt	+	+ + +	+		+		
Copper					+		
Germanium	+		+		+		
Lead		+ + +	+ + +		+	+ + +	+
Lithium		+ +	+ +				
Mercury	+	+ + +	+ +	+		+ + +	
Molybdenum		+		+			
Nickel	+ +	+			+		
Platinum			+				
Rubidium							
Selenium				+			
Strontium							
Vanadium	+	+	+			+	+
Zinc							+

spectrum of toxicity, with the nature and severity being dependent on the chemical form and oxidation state of the arsenical involved. Arsine, a compound that binds tightly to erythrocytes, causes hemolysis and subsequent renal damage that persists following a single acute exposure.[7] The trivalent and pentavalent arsenicals represent decreased orders of toxicity, as the latter is more readily excreted and constitutes the most common environmental form.[4] Nonetheless, all compounds produce inhibition of sulfhydryl enzymes and can uncouple mitochondrial oxidase phosphorylation resulting in the inhibition of cellular respiration. In most chronic forms of arsenic intoxication, gastrointestinal disturbances, skin pigmentation, anemia, and disturbances in hepatic and neurological function may occur. Electrocardiographic changes have also been observed in arsenic poisoned patients[8,9,10] whose serum electrolytes (potassium) were normal, suggesting that arsenic was exerting a direct toxic effect on the myocardium.

ANTIMONY. The symptoms of acute and chronic antimony compounds are similar to those caused by arsenic, and toxic effects are elicited more frequently by the trivalent than by the pentavalent compounds.[11] Antimony compounds are powerful emetics by virtue of their irritant effects on the intestinal tract. Antimony compounds can also cause pronounced vasodilator effects on the circulatory system resulting in a shock-like syndrome. Electrocardiographic studies, in patients treated with trivalent antimonials for schistosomiasis, have revealed significant changes during therapy in a high percentage of patients,[12,13] and some authors have reviewed these changes as indicative of direct myocardial damage.[13,14]

MERCURY. Mercury compounds combine with the sulfhydryl groups of enzymes and proteins, and it is this effect that accounts for most of the biological properties of the metal.[15] Mercury intoxication generally affects the mouth, colon, and kidney. Acute ingestion produces a stomatitis with metallic taste often accompanied by an ashen-gray discoloration of the pharynx, anemia, and gastrointestinal disturbances. Pure mercury poses a hazard because of its volatility, and absorption by inhalation of fumes produces pneumonitis and other respiratory complications. All mercury compounds depress tubular mechanisms in the kidney, responsible for the active reabsorption of sodium and chloride; however, unlike organic mercurials that are rapidly excreted, inorganic mercury compounds accumulate and can produce extensive functional damage. At higher levels of exposure, the central nervous system is affected leading to serious and frequently permanent damage. Because of their greater lipid solubility, organic mercuric compounds (methyl mercury) can produce profound neurological effects. The nervous condition of hatters throughout the early nineteenth century was due to chronic exposure to mercury that was used to soften felt.[1] Mercury has also been shown to cause embryopathic and teratogenic effects in animals, and to induce fetal toxicity in mothers undergoing mercurial therapy.

LEAD. Lead intoxication is a progressive process, and toxic effects are often dose related. Chronic exposure to low concentrations of lead decreases heme biosynthesis, affecting the production of hemoglobin and red blood cells. Impairment of the enzymes delta-aminolevulinic acid (ALA) synthetase, ALA dehydrase (ALA-d), coproporphyrinogen oxidase, and heme synthetase by sulfhydryl inhibition is responsible for the anemia of lead poisoning.[2] The ALA-d activity may be the most sensitive biological parameter of lead effect that is presently measurable,[16] and it has been established that a progressive inhibition of this enzyme is found with increasing blood lead concentrations. The activity of this enzyme is inhibited in lead-exposed experimental animals, in workers exposed to lead as a result of their occupation, and in lead poisoned children.[2] The measurement of the enzyme activity in circulating red blood cells is a sensitive index of lead poisoning and has been used to screen children for the disease. Another early sign of lead poisoning is acute abdominal colic, which usually develops when the blood lead concentration reaches 80 ug/dl, a concentration that has generally been accepted as the threshold for indicating clinical poisoning.[2] Chronic exposure to lead will eventually produce a line of deep-blue pigmentation in the gingival margin due to the precipitation of lead sulphide, and, upon radiological examination, the presence of a lead line (increased radio-density) at the growing ends (epiphyseal portions) of long bones will be evident. The large deposition of lead into bones was once thought to represent a detoxification mechanism; however, certain conditions such as metabolic acidosis can mobilize lead to more susceptible tissues. At higher levels of exposure, acute encephalopathy, the most serious manifestation of lead poisoning characterized by convulsions and coma, and renal complications can occur.

CADMIUM. Cadmium has industrial applications such as electroplating, pigment production, and the manufacture of plastics, a number of which can result in environmental contamination. Without specific recognized exposures, the kidney is considered to be the critical organ for cadmium accumulation, and the renal cortex contains one-third of the total body content. While little is present at birth, cadmium accumulates in the kidneys during the first two decades of life, rising to a value of 10 mgs of renal cadmium for the average American adult. Cadmium concentrations in other tissues including lung are low; although, acute cadmium exposure produces pulmonary toxicity, such as swelling and hyperplasia of bronchial cells, leading to chronic pneumonitis.[17] In 1960, purification of a cadmium binding protein from equine kidneys was reported by Kagi and Valloo.[18] Metallothionein, a low molecular weight protein of 10,000, has been found in the human kidney in amounts sufficient to account for all of the cadmium concentrated in this organ. It is generally accepted that the calcium loss via the kidney damaged by cadmium was responsible for the bone deformities in Itai-itai disease.[19] One epidemiological study has suggested a relationship between human exposure and renal cancer,[20] and cadmium has been shown to be carcinogenic in rodents;[21] although, the carcinogenic effects of cadmium are controversial.

While heavy metal intoxication usually results in generalized syndromes involving many organs, several metals can exhibit more discrete toxic effects.[17] The most common signs of exposure to beryllium are skin lesions such as dermatitis, ulceration, and granulomas. These lesions often occur after a long latent period in conjunction with the chronic pulmonary aspect of beryllium intoxication. Polycythemia is the characteristic response of most mammals, including man, to ingestion of large amounts of cobalt and has been used in the treatment of refractory anemias. Vanadium selectively produces pulmonary toxicity, and most of the clinical symptoms observed following industrial exposures reflect its irritant effects on the respiratory system. Recent studies have shown that vanadium salts are quite toxic for alveolar macrophages *in vitro*,[22] which are known to be important in pulmonary defense, suggesting that vanadium may predispose the exposed individual to pulmonary infections. Finally, epidemiological studies have suggested that certain occupational exposures of workmen to chromium and nickel are associated with an increased incidence of certain types of tumors, and compounds of seven metals (beryllium, cadmium, chromium, cobalt, lead, nickel, and zinc) have been shown to induce cancer in experimental animals.[21]

Low Level Exposure

The broad utilization of heavy metals and consequent distribution into the general environment raises the issue of possible chronic exposure and low level intoxication. This section will deal with the relationship between cadmium and cardiovascular disease, especially hypertension, and the possible subtle effects of lead (especially in young animals and children) on cardiovascular and behavioral development, when classical signs of lead intoxication are absent. There is considerable logic in studying the definative role of metals in hypertension, because a large number of anti-hypertensive drugs (nitroprusside) have the common ability to bind transitional and related trace elements.[23] Also, epidemological studies have suggested a relationship between heavy metal intoxication and cardiovascular abnormalities.

Kobayasski[24] initially suggested that some types of cardiovascular disease might be related to water quality, and this association might explain some of the geographical variations in the incidence of certain cardiovascular diseases. Many epidemiological studies have shown that the incidence of cardiovascular disease, including hypertension and ischemic heart disease, is higher in soft water areas when compared to hard water ones.[2,25] Soft water is slightly acidic due to carbon dioxide dissolved in it from air and from decaying organisms that occur naturally in reservoirs and can corrode metal pipes. Conversely, hard water contains calcium and magnesium bicarbonates, which precipitate on metal pipes forming a hard coating that can resist corrosion. It has been suggested that the inverse relationship between cardiovascular disease and the hardness of water might be explained by the leaching of cadmium or lead from its source material by soft water. This reasoning has stimulated a search for signs of increased heavy metal absorption in persons dying from cardiovascular diseases; however, the association of hypertension with high kidney levels of cadmium in certain studies is not sufficient to establish a cause and effect relationship.

CADMIUM. Cadmium is an especially likely candidate for an association with hypertension because of the affinity of this metal for the kidney, an organ known to be involved in blood pressure regulation. One study has shown that cadmium-exposed workers have high renal cadmium levels if they do not have renal failure, but have low levels when renal failure has occurred.[19] Because of the severe renal impairment, this observation may explain why patients suffering from Itai-itai disease did not exhibit hypertension or high renal cadmium concentrations. Schroeder[26] related blood pressure to renal cadmium concentration in American accident victims, and found that hypertensive subjects had more renal cadmium than normotensive controls. In a similar study using living patients, untreated hypertensive patients exhibited higher blood cadmium levels than a matched group of untreated controls.[27] These studies suggest that cadmium, at levels that are not nephrotoxic, may be involved in the genesis of hypertension.

Perhaps the strongest evidence linking cadmium to hypertension is that ingestion of extremely small quantities of cadmium by rodents produces a significant increase in blood pressure. In an initial study, Schroeder[28] found that rats, chronically exposed to 0.0005 percent (or 5 ppm) cadmium in drinking water, develop hypertension with systolic pressures that were more than 35 mm Hg above the mean value for age-matched control animals. The significant increase in blood pressure in exposed animals occurred in the absence of the usual toxic manifestations associated with more intensive cadmium exposure. This blood pressure response was a specific effect of low level cadmium exposure, since the administration of other metals (such as vanadium, chromium, nickel, arsenic, selenium, antimony, and lead) at similar concentrations did not promote the development of hypertension.[1] Other investigators have confirmed the induction of hypertension by chronic cadmium feeding, and have reported statistically significant increases in blood pressure after one month of exposure.[29] A recent study has shown that exposure of rats to 0.10 to 5.0 ppm cadmium in drinking water produces a relatively constant blood pressure increase of 15 to 20 mm Hg.[30] Although cadmium induced hypertension in rats seems to be relatively small in magnitude, this effect mimics the insidious pathology associated with essential hypertension in humans. Survival of cadmium-exposed rats with hypertension was less than survival among control animals, suggesting that as in man, hypertension was associated with an increased mortality rate.[31] Moreover, cadmium fed rats accumulated renal concentrations of the metal that were similar to those of hypertensive humans with inapparent exposure. Cadmium-induced hypertension has also been produced in rabbits[32] and dogs.[33]

Although the mechanism of cadmium-induced hypertension in animals is not well defined, several possible mechanisms have been suggested. In acute hypertension induced by parental cadmium injection, the immediate increase in blood pressure can be directly related to an increase in cardiac output.[34] Cadmium ingestion in rats produced chronic hypertension that is accompanied by an increase in circulating renin.[35,36] Finally, cadmium administration to rats has been shown to promote sodium retention.[37]

The effects of drugs in cadmium-induced hypertension has also been investigated. Hypertensive rats, given 10 ppm cadmium in drinking water, have depressed responses to norepinephrine and angiotensin, which is similar to the diminished vascular reactivity that is characteristic of some types of human hypertension.[38] The vascular reactivity of aortic strips from cadmium-injected hypertensive rabbits exhibited a decreased responsiveness to angiotensin, but not to norepinephrine.[32] A recent study has shown; however, that cadmium may either increase or reduce the pressor response to norepinephrine in rats, and this effect is dose-related.[39] Exposure to cadmium at levels that do not produce overt hypertension cause a potentiation of the pressor response to norepinephrine, and this effect wears off with time if exposure is discontinued. Studies using isolated vessels (aorta and tail artery) suggest that sensitization of the arteries to adrenergic stimulation is probably the mechanism by which low level cadmium exposure potentiates the norepinephrine pressor response.[39] Rats chronically exposed to higher cadmium concentrations exhibit normal growth and hypertension initially; however, these animals eventually develop hypotension possibly resulting from extensive renal impairment.[30]

While the causes of essential human hypertension remain unknown, the possible relationship between environmental factors and human hypertension warrants further investigation. Many studies have shown that ingestion or injection of low cadmium concentrations can induce hypertension in animals. It must be emphasized, however, that heavy (or high level) cadmium exposure is not associated with hypertension in animals or man. Rats exposed to high concentrations of cadmium in drinking water (50 ppm) exhibit hypertension only during the early portion of exposure before overt toxicity becomes evident.[30] In man, Itai-itai disease and chronic cadmium poisoning is not associated with high blood pressure. If cadmium plays any part in human hypertension, it is probably early in the course of this disease. Although it is evident that cadmium is an ubiquitous environmental contaminant that is sometimes present in concentrations that can induce hypertension in rats, the extent, if any, to which these observations can be extrapolated from animals to man remains to be determined. Consequently, it appears necessary to minimize cadmium exposure as much as economically feasible until future studies clarify the possible relationship between exposure and human hypertension.

LEAD. Within the last several years, the atmospheric concentration of lead has been estimated to be increasing at a faster rate than any other metal pollutant. While federal regulation regarding lead additives in gasoline promises to slow the rate of increase, lead in the environment will remain a significant health hazard due to the possibility of low level human exposure. Although the effects of acute and chronic exposure to high concentrations of lead have been well studied, the detrimental effects associated with long term exposure to low concentrations of lead are not well understood. These effects are produced by exposure to lead at concentrations too low to produce the symptoms commonly associated with lead toxicity, and have been termed *subclinical* due to the absence of the classical signs of lead intoxication.[2] This type of intoxication has been associated with peripheral neuropathy in lead workers[40] and abnormalities in erythrocyte function.[41] Some behavioral and neuropsychological disorders have also been suggested to occur as latent sequelae of increased lead absorption in children.[42,43] There is need to establish whether present-day environmental levels of lead are capable of producing harmful physiological or psychological effects in children who are most at risk. Many studies have indicated that children and young animals[44] are more susceptible to toxic effects of lead than adults. Threshold levels for anemia and neurological impairment due to lead exposure are lower for children than adults.[45]

Many investigators have used the suckling rat as a model of chronic lead toxicity. Pentschew and Garro[46] fed lead carbonate to dams and observed the development of an encephalopathy in suckling rats that was comparable to the pathology of lead intoxication in children. This effect occurred despite the lack of observable toxicity in the mother, illustrating the great difference in the sensitivity of the suckling and mature rats to the central effects of lead. By reducing the lead concentration in the maternal diet, other investigators[47,48] have found that chronic lead exposure of rodents (via dam's milk) produced pups who had no overt signs of pathology but showed a marked increase in motor activity. Although exposed pups grew at a slower rate than did controls and malnutrition alone can produce similar behavioral changes,[49] behavioral effects have been observed in lead-exposed rats who exhibited no growth retardation.[50,51,52]

In addition to hyperactivity, lead treatment has also been shown to impair learning ability in rats.[53] This study showed not only that lead exposure of suckling rats causes decreases in learning ability, but also that days one to ten after parturition were critical in the production of this effect of lead. Administration of lead to dams throughout the twenty-one day nursing period caused decreased learning ability in eight to ten week old offspring. A similar effect was seen when lead was administered to dams on days one through ten, but not days eleven through twenty-one of the nursing period. Significant in this study was the observation that blood lead levels had decreased to control when the impaired learning ability was observed. Presumably, exposure to lead shortly after birth produced some degree of central nervous system dysfunction that persisted in adult animals.

Various clinical observations indicate an involvement of lead in the pathogenesis of cardiovascular disease. Patients dying from coronary artery disease in soft water areas were found to have higher bone lead levels than those from hard water areas.[54] Beevers and co-workers[55] have shown a positive correlation between an increased incidence of hypertension and elevated blood lead levels. Electrocardiographic abnormalities[56,57] and atrio-ventricular conduction defects[58] have been observed in humans suffering from lead intoxication. A reversible myocarditis in patients with documented lead intoxication has been observed in several instances.[59,60] While no clear relationship between lead exposure and cardiovascular disease has emerged, enough observation of cardiac involvement has been made to warrant careful study of these effects.

An alteration in the function of the automatic nervous system might produce some of the behavioral and cardiovascular disturbances observed during chronic lead intoxication. Lead added *in vitro* has been shown to inhibit synaptic transmission and reduce acetylcholine output in the perfused superior cervical ganglion of the cat.[61] Chronic lead exposure in rodents has been shown to produce enhanced adrenergic function and diminished cholinergic function in the central nervous system.[62] The hyperactivity reported in rats after neonatal lead exposure probably results from an alteration in central autonomic function, since this abnormality could be suppressed by adrenergic antagonists and exacerbated by cholinergic antagonists.[63] An increased urinary excretion of catecholamine metabolites has also been reported after chronic lead exposure in mice and in children with increased lead absorption.[64] Electrocardiographic changes in lead-fed dogs were suggested to result, at least in part, from disturbances in the function of the autonomic nervous system.[65] Cardiac disturbances in lead-poisoned humans possibly resulting from increased vagal tone include bradycardia,[56] heart block,[58] and marked sinus depression with multiple ventricular extrasystoles.[66]

Relatively few experimental studies have examined the effects of lead on cardiovascular function. Rats given water containing lead were shown to develop biochemical and morphological changes in cardiac muscle.[67] Myocardial changes observed included an increased deposition of lead in the heart, a reduction in the activity of certain cardiac enzymes (ferrochelatase and deltaaminoleavulinic acid dehydrase), and marked electron microscopic changes in cardiac muscle. While epidemiological studies have suggested that lead exposure might be a causative factor in promoting hypertension in humans, prolonged administration of lead to rats has produced no significant change in mean arterial blood pressure.[68]

While cardiovascular abnormalities have been observed in adults suffering from symptomatic lead poisoning,[66] little is known concerning the cardiac effects of chronic exposure early in life.[59,60] Our studies have examined cardiac function in adult rats exposed to lead for only the first twenty-one days of life. One function of the autonomic nervous system is the cardiovascular reflex control of circulation, and, since lead can produce autonomic dysfunction, a period of lead exposure was selected that would coincide with the development of adrenergic innervation.[69]

Suckling rats were exposed according to the method described by Bornschein et al., when, upon parturition, dams were given a 0.2 percent lead acetate solution substituted for drinking water.[70] Hence, newborn rats were chronically exposed to lead via mother's milk from birth to weaning. Mothers of control litters were supplied a sodium acetate solution. Lead was readily conveyed to the suckling rats, as dams given 0.2 percent lead acetate had blood lead levels of 65 ± 6 ug/dl and their pups had blood lead levels of 47 ± 3 *ug/dl* on the final day of nursing.[71] Control blood lead levels were 4 ± 3 1 and 6 ± 1 ug/dl, respectively. A significant concentration of lead also accumulated in the heart of exposed pups (4.0 ± 0.12 *vs* 0.5 ± 0.10 ug/g wet weight for control) during the twenty-one day treatment period. Cardiovascular experiments were performed using rats four months of age.

Norepinephrine was given to test the responsiveness of the cardiovascular system, because of the importance of this compound in blood pressure control and adrenergic neurotransmission.[72] Mean arterial blood pressure of lead-exposed animals was no different from that of control, and increases in blood pressure produced by injection of 1, 5, and 10 ug/kg of norepinephrine were the same in both groups of animals. Although cardiac arrhythmias were observed in only a few of the control animals and only after the higher doses of norepinephrine, all doses of the catecholamine caused the appearance of ventricular extrasystoles in lead-exposed animals. Doses of norepinephrine that caused no significant electrocardiographic abnormalities in control animals were arrhythmogenic in lead-exposed animals.

Since the only striking difference between lead-exposed and control animals in these initial studies was in the generation of cardiac arrhythmias, experiments were performed in which norepinephrine was administered in a manner known to produce cardiac rhythm disturbances. The effect of norepinephrine on the electrocardiogram (standard limb lead II) of lead-exposed and control animals is shown in Figure 4–1. A two minute i.v. infusion of norepinephrine (80 ug/kg min^{-1}) caused a small number of cardiac arrhythmias in all control animals tested. Several different alterations in the electrocardiogram occurred, ranging from S-T segment depression to ventricular tachycardia, but ventricular extrasystoles (or premature beats) were the most consistently observed disturbance in cardiac rhythm. Therefore, the number of extrasystoles occurring during a two minute infusion period was taken as a measure of arrhythmogenic activity. Infusion of norepinephrine produced more than four times as many ventricular extrasystoles in lead-exposed rats than in age-matched control animals (Figure 4–2).

The mechanism of the altered norepinephrine response produced by neonatal lead exposure has been investigated.[73,74] Two factors were identified that singly or in combination could lead to the enhanced sensitivity of lead-exposed rats to the arrhythmogenic action of norepinephrine. Norepinephrine has effects directly on the heart and indirectly via reflex vagal stimulation, both of which could conceivably produce cardiac rhythm disturbances. Further experiments have indicated that the direct cardiac effects and the indirect reflex vagal effects of norepinephrine are both involved in the arrhythmogenic responses of lead-exposed animals. Bilateral vagotomy or atropine pretreatment before infusion of norepinephrine (Fig. 4–2) significantly decreased the frequency of

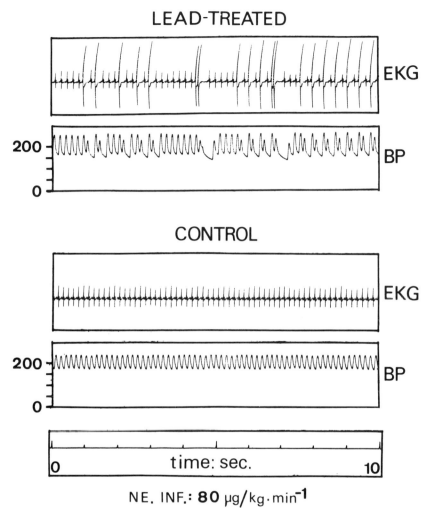

Figure 4–1. Effect of norepinephrine infusion on the electrocardiogram and blood pressure (polygraph) tracings taken from adult lead-exposed and control rats.

cardiac arrhythmias; although, norepinephrine still caused significantly more ventricular extrasystoles in lead-exposed animals than control. A two minute infusion of methoxamine (800 ug/ kg min^{-1}) also produced significantly more ventricular extrasystoles in lead-exposed rats than in control. But this response could be completely prevented by bilateral vagotomy prior to infusion, indicating cardiac effects of this drug were mediated

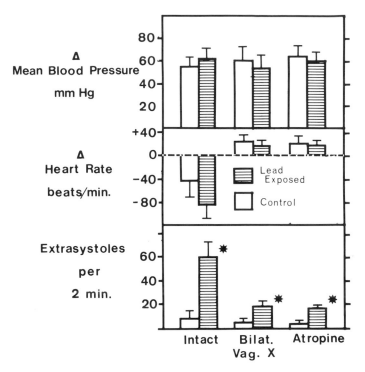

Figure 4–2. The effect of norepinephrine in lead-exposed and control rats before and after bilateral vagotomy or atropine administration (1 mg/kg). Rats were exposed to 0.2 percent lead acetate via maternal milk during the twenty-one day nursing period. Preinjection blood pressures and heart rates of lead-exposed and control rats in each experimental group were not significantly different. Blood pressure and heart rate are shown as maximum changes during the two minute infusion period. Stars denote responses in lead-exposed animals that significantly differ from control.

through the large increase in mean systemic blood pressure and the subsequent reflex vagal activity. Isolated, perfused, spontaneously beating rat hearts from lead-exposed rats also exhibited more irregularities in cardiac rhythm after norepinephrine administration than did hearts from control animals (Figure 4–3). These experiments indicate that while vagal reflex effects participate in the lead induced sensitivity to norepinephrine, direct cardiac effects are also involved.

Other experiments were performed to study the relationship of the time and level of exposure to the extent of cardiotoxicity

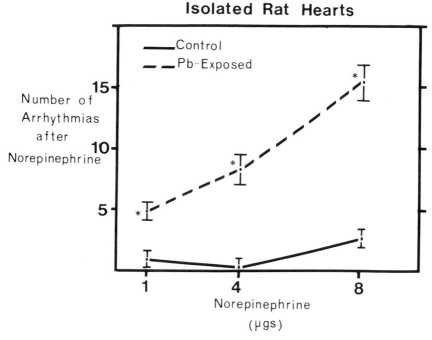

Isolated Rat Hearts

Figure 4–3. Arrhythmogenic responses of isolated, perfused, spontaneously beat-ing rat hearts to graded doses of norepinephrine. The basal heart rates and contractile tension of isolated hearts taken from lead-exposed and control rats were not significantly different from control. Extrasystoles were the most common cardiac rhythm disturbance observed in either group. Asterisks denote responses in lead-exposed animals that significantly differ from control.

produced.[75] Since it had been shown that pups nursed by dams receiving 0.2 percent lead acetate solution exhibited an abnormal cardiac response to norepinephrine, lead solutions of lower con-centrations (0.1 % and 0.05 %) were tested. Only rats whose dams were exposed to 0.2 percent lead acetate exhibited the increased sensitivity to norepinephrine, indicating that the level of lead exposure required to produce norepinephrine cardiotoxicity was quite narrow.

In another series, rats were exposed to lead as described previously, except that instead of receiving lead solution through-out the entire nursing period, dams received 0.2 percent lead acetate days one to ten or eleven through twenty-one only.[75]

Norepinephrine produced significantly more ventricular arrhythmias in adult rats from litters exposed to 0.2 percent lead
from days one through ten than control (Figure 4–4). Rats exposed
to comparable levels of lead exposure during days eleven through
twenty-one responded to norepinephrine in a manner no different
from control. Moreover, the number of cardiac rhythm disturbances observed in rats exposed to lead from days one to ten did not
differ significantly from those exposed to the same lead level from
days one to twenty-one (Fig. 4–2). The responses of animals in both
lead exposure groups to bilateral vagotomy before the infusion of
norepinephrine was also similar. Also shown in Figure 4–4, rats
exposed to lead for only the first ten days of nursing accumulated
43 percent of the cardiac lead concentration and 80 percent of the
blood lead concentration obtained in rats exposed for the entire
twenty-one day nursing period. Tissue lead accumulation during
the first ten days of life is critical for the development of this
cardiac abnormality.

Since adrenergic development occurs at a time when the cardiac
sensitivity to lead is most pronounced, the endogenous norepinephrine concentration was measured during this time period
as an index of functional innervation. Early exposure to lead at
levels that are known to produce norepinephrine cardiotoxicity
produced a 50 percent decrease in the endogenous ventricular
norepinephrine content.[76] These results suggest that early exposure to lead might produce adrenergic nerve terminal lesions in
the heart by altering the course of normal adrenergic development. A deficiency or unevenness of adrenergic innervation may
predispose these animals to the arrhythmogenic effects of norepinephrine.

Since all foregoing experiments were performed using rats at
least four months of age, it was decided to test the response of rats
of different ages to norepinephrine infusion.[77]

As shown in Figure 4–5, the incidence of norepinephrine induced
cardiac arrhythmias (ventricular extrasystoles) increases with age
in control animals. The norepinephrine content of the heart is
known to decrease and the incidence of certain cardiac arrhythmias
has been shown to increase with ageing in rats and other animals.
The regression lines indicate that this relationship is augmented

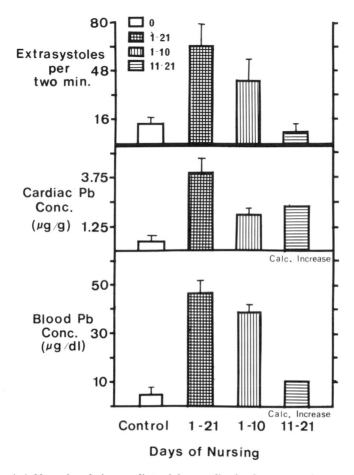

Figure 4–4. Norepinephrine cardiotoxicity, cardiac lead concentrations, and blood lead levels in relation to the time of lead exposure during the nursing period. Lactating dams were treated with 0.2 percent lead acetate in drinking water during the time periods denoted. Cardiac and blood lead concentrations were determined in animals twenty-one days of age (final day of nursing), while arrhythmogenic responses to norepinephrine were tested in rats four months of age. Only rats exposed to 0.2 percent lead during the first ten days of nursing exhibited significantly more ventricular extrasystoles than control.

in lead-exposed animals, due to subtle developmental changes that occur during the first ten days of life. If this cardiotoxicity seen in rats occurs in a similar fashion in humans, low level lead

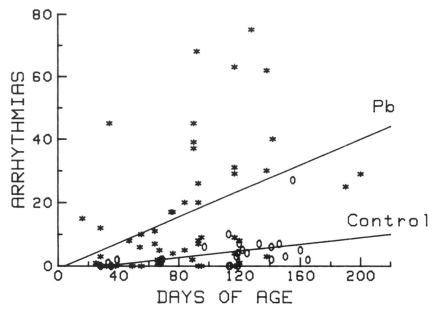

Figure 4–5. Infusion of norepinephrine in lead-exposed (0.2%) and control rats of different ages (26 to 200 days of life). Lines for both groups were determined by linear regression analysis, and the slopes differ significantly. Each line represents data obtained from thirty to fifty-four animals in either group.

exposure in children might produce adults with a high risk of cardiac disease. Further studies in this area could help define the role of environmental factors in heart disease.

REFERENCES

1. Schroeder, H. A.: *The Trace Elements and Man; Some Positive and Negative Aspects.* Old Greenwich, Devin-Adair Co., 1973.
2. Waldron, H. A. and Stofen, D.: *Subclinical Lead Poisoning.* New York City, Academic Press Inc., 1974.
3. Kestaloot, H., Roelandt, J., Williams, J., Claes, J. H., and Joossens, J. V.: An inquiry into the role of cobalt in the heart disease of chronic beer drinkers. *Cir, 37:*854–864, 1968.
4. Fowler, B. A.: Toxicology of environmental arsenic. In Goyer, R. A. and Mehlman, M. A. (Eds.): *Toxicology of Trace Elements.* Washington, D. C., Hemisphere Publ. Co., 1977. pp. 79–122.
5. D'Itri, R. M.: *The Environmental Mercury Problem.* Cleveland, CRC Press, 1972.
6. Beliles, R. B.: Metals. In Casarett, L. J. and Doull, J. (Eds.): *Toxicology (The*

Basic Science of Poisons). New York City, Macmillan Publ. Co., Inc., 1975. p. 457.

7. Fowler, B. A. and Weissberg, J. B.: Arsine Poisoning. *New Eng J Med, 291:*1171–1174, 1974.

8. Josephson, C. J., Pinto, S. S., and Petronella, S. J.: Arsine: electrocardiographic changes produced in acute human poisoning. *Arch Ind Hyg Occup Med, 4:*43–53, 1951.

9. Barry, K. G. and Herndon, E. G., Jr.: Electrocardiographic changes associated with acute arsenic poisoning. *Med Ann DC, 31:*65–66, 1962.

10. Glazener, F. S., Ellis, J. G., and Johnson, P. K.: Electrocardiographic findings with arsenic poisoning. *Calif Med, 109:*158–162, 1968.

11. Harvey, S. C.: Heavy Metals. In Goodman, L. S. and Gillman, A. F. (Eds.): *The Pharmacological Basis of Therapeutics.* New York City, Macmillan Publ. Co., Inc., 1975, pp. 924–945.

12. O'Brien, W.: The effect of antimony on the heart. *Trans Roy Soc Trop Med Hyg, 53:*482–486, 1959.

13. Honey, M.: The effects of sodium antimony tartrate on the myocardium. *Brit Heart J, 22:*601–616, 1960.

14. Mainzer, F., and Krause, M.: Changes in the electrocardiogram appearing during antimony treatment. *Trans Roy Soc Trop Med Hyg, 33:*405–418, 1940.

15. Clarkson, T. W.: The pharmacology of mercurial compounds. *Ann Rev Pharmacol, 12:*375–406, 1972.

16. Haeger-Aronsen, B., Abdulla, M., and Fristedt, B. I.: Effect of lead on –aminolevulinic acid dehydrase activity in red blood cells. *Arch Environ Health, 23:*440–445, 1971.

17. Hennigar, G. R.: Drug and chemical injury. In Anderson, W. A. (Ed.): *Pathology.* St. Louis, C. V. Mosby Co., 1971, pp. 174–241.

18. Kagi, J. H. and Valloo, B. L.: A cadmium– and zinc-containing protein from equine renal cortex. *J Biol Chem, 236:*2435–2442, 1961.

19. Friberg, I., Piscator, M., and Nordberg, G.: *Cadmium in the Environment.* Cleveland, CRC Press, 1971.

20. Kolonel, L. N.: Association of cadmium with renal cancer. *Cancer, 37:*1782–1787, 1976.

21. Sunderman, F. W., Jr.: Metal carcinogenesis. In Goyer, R. A. and Mehlman, M. A. (Eds.): *Toxicology of Trace Elements.* Washington, D.C., Hemisphere Publ. Co., 1977. pp. 257–285.

22. Waters, M. D., Gardner, D. E., and Coffin, D. L.: Cytotoxic effects of vanadium on rabbit alveolar macrophages *in vitro. Toxicol. Appl. Pharmacol., 28:*253–263, 1974.

23. Perry, H. M., Jr.: Hypertension and the geochemical environment. *Ann N Y Acad Sci, 199:*202–215, 1972.

24. Kobayashi, J.: Geographical relationship between chemical nature of river water and death-rate from apoplexy. *Benchete Ohara Inst Landivertsch Biologie, 11:*12–22, 1957.

25. Schroeder, H. A.: Relation between mortality from cardiovascular disease

and treated water supplies. *JAMA, 172:*1902–1908, 1960.

26. Schroeder, H. A.: Cadmium as a factor in hypertension. *J Chronic Dis, 18:*217–228, 1965.

27. Glauser, S. C., Bello, C. T., and Glauser, E. M.: Blood-cadmium levels in normotensive and hypertensive humans. *Lancet, 1:*717–718, 1976.

28. Schroeder, H. A.: Cadmium hypertension in rats. *Amer J Physiol, 207:*62–66, 1964.

29. Perry, H. M., Jr. and Erlanger, M. W.: Hypertension in rats induced by long-term low-level cadmium ingestion. *Cir, 40:*130, 1971.

30. Perry, H. M., Erlanger, M., and Perry, E. F.: Increase in systolic blood pressure of rats chronically fed cadmium. *Environ Health Persp, 28:*251–260, 1973.

31. Schroeder, H. A., Kroll, B. A., Little, J. W., Livingston, P. O. and Myers, M.: Hypertension in rats from injection of cadmium. *Arch Environ Health, 13:*788–789, 1966.

32. Thind, G. S., Karreman, G., Stephan, K. F., and Blakemore, W. S.: Vascular reactivity and mechanical properties of normal and cadmium-hypertensive rabbits. *J Lab Clin Med, 76:*560–568, 1970.

33. Thind, G. S., Biery, D. N., and Bovee, K. C.: Production of arterial hypertension by cadmium in dog. *J Lab Clin Med, 81:*549–556, 1973.

34. Perry, H. M., Jr., Erlanger, M., Yunice, A., and Perry, E. F.: Mechanism of the acute hypertensive effect of intra-arterial cadmium and mercury in anesthetized rats. *J Lab Clin Med, 70:*963–972, 1967.

35. Perry, H. M., Jr. and Erlanger, M. W.: Elevated peripheral renin activity in cadmium-induced hypertension. *J Lab Clin Med, 76:*852–853, 1970.

36. Perry, H. M., Jr. and Erlanger, M. W.: Elevated circulating renin activity in rats following doses of cadmium known to induce hypertension. *J Lab Clin Med, 82:*339–405, 1973.

37. Perry, H. M., Jr., Perry, E. F., and Purifoy, J. E.: Antinatriuretic effect of intramuscular cadmium in rats. *Proc Soc Exp Biol Med, 136:*1240–1248, 1971.

38. Schroeder, H. A., Baker, J. T., Hansen, Jr., N. M., Size, J. G., and Wise, R. A.: Vascular reactivity of rats altered by cadmium and a zinc chelate. *Arch Environ Health, 21:*609–614, 1970.

39. Nechay, B. R., Williams, B. J., Steinsland, O. S., and Hall, C. E.: Increased vascular responses to adrenergic stimulation in rats exposed to cadmium. *J Toxicol Environ Health, 4:*559–567, 1978.

40. Seppalainen, A. M., Tola, S., Hernberg, S., and Kock, B.: Subclinical neuropathy at safe levels of lead exposure. *Arch Environ Health, 30:*180–183, 1975.

41. Sakuri, K., Suguta, M., and Tsuchiya, K.: Biological response and subjective symptoms in low level lead exposure. *Arch Environ Health, 29:*157–163, 1974.

42. David, O., Clark, J., and Voeller, J.: Lead and hyperactivity. *Lancet, 2:*900–903, 1972.

43. dela Burde, B. and Choate, M. S., Jr.: Does asymptomatic lead exposure in children have latent sequela? *J Pediatr, 81:*1088–1091, 1972.
44. Sharding, N. N. and Oehme, F. W.: The use of animal models for comparative studies of lead poisoning. *Clin Toxicol Bull, 3:*104–110, 1973.
45. Lamola, A. A., Joselow, M., and Yamane, T.: Zinc protoporphyrin: a simple sensitive fluorometric screening test for lead poisoning. *Clin Chem, 21:*93–97, 1975.
46. Pentschew, A. and Garro, F.: Lead encephalo-myelopathy of the suckling rat and its implications on the porphyrinopathic nervous diseases. *Acta Neuropathologica, 6:*266–278, 1966.
47. Silbergeld, E. K. and Goldberg, A. M.: A lead-induced behavioral disorder. *Life Sci, 13:*1375–1383, 1973.
48. Sauerhoff, M. W. and Michaelson, I. A.: Hyperactivity and brain catecholamines in lead-exposed developing rats. *Science, 182:*1022–1024, 1973.
49. Loch, R., Bornschein, R. L., and Michaelson, I. A.: Role of undernutrition in the paradoxical response of lead-exposed hyperactive mice to amphetamine and phenobarbital. *Pharmacol, 18:*124, 1976.
50. Golter, M. and Michaelson, I. A.: Growth, behavior, and brain catecholamines in lead-exposed neonatal rats: a reappraisal. *Science, 187:*359–361, 1975.
51. Wince, L. C., Donovan, C. H., and Azzero, A. J.: Behavioral and biochemical analysis of the lead-exposed hyperactive rat. *Pharmacol, 18:*198, 1976.
52. Overmann, S. R.: Behavioral effects of asymptomatic lead exsure during neonatal development in rats. *Toxicol Appl Pharmacol, 41:*459–471, 1977.
53. Brown, D. R.: Neonatal lead exposure in the rat: decreased learning as a function of age and blood lead concentration. *Toxicol and Appl Pharmacol, 32:*628–637, 1975.
54. Crawford, D. and Crawford, T.: Lead content of bones in a soft and hard water area. *Lancet, 1:*699–701, 1969.
55. Beevers, D. G., Erskine, E., and Robertson, M.: Blood-lead and hypertension. *Lancet, 2:*1–3, 1976.
56. Read, J. L. and Williams, J. P.: Lead myocarditis, report of a case. *Amer Heart J, 44:*797–802, 1952.
57. Kosmider, S. and Pentelenz, T.: Zmiany electrokardiograficzne u starszych osob z przewlekym sawodowym zatrucien olowiem. *Pol Arch Med, 32:*437–442, 1962.
58. Myerson, R. M. and Eisenhauer, J. H.: Atrioventricular conduction defects in lead poisoning. *Amer J Cardiol, 11:*409–413, 1963.
59. Freeman, R.: Reversible myocarditis due to chronic lead poisoning in childhood. *Arch Dis Child, 40:*389–393, 1965.
60. Kline, T. S.: Myocardial changes in lead poisoning. *Amer J Dis Child, 99:*48–54, 1960.
61. Kostial, K. and Vouk, V. B.: Lead ions and synaptic transmission in the superior cervical ganglia of the cat. *Brit J Pharmacol, 12:*219–222, 1957.
62. Shih, T. M. and Hanin, T.: Chronic lead exposure in immature rodents, neurochemical correlates. *Life Sci, 23:*877–888, 1978.

63. Silbergeld, E. K. and Goldberg, A. M.: Pharmacological and neurochemical investigations of lead-induced hyperactivity. *Neuropharmacol, 14:*431–444, 1975.

64. Silbergeld, E. K. and Chisholm, J. J.: Lead poisoning: altered urinary catecholamine metabolites as indicators of intoxication in mice and men. *Science, 192:*153–155, 1976.

65. Stykhinskaya, M. I.: Elektrokardiograficheskic izmeneniyz ped khronicheskim na zhivotnye deistuiem svintsa. *Trud Kazak Inst Patol Akad Medit, 14:*56–60, 1965.

66. Crepet, M., Gobbato, F., and Scansetti, G.: Le alterazioni cardiovascolari nei lavoratori del piombo. *Min Med, 47:*1910–1918, 1956.

67. Moore, M. R., Goldberg, A., Carr, K., Toner, P., and Lawrie, T. D. V.: Biochemical and electro-microscopical studies of chronic lead exposure in the heart and other organs of rats. *Scot Med J, 19:*155–156, 1974.

68. Padilla, F, Shapiro, A. P., and Jensen, W. N.: Effect of chronic lead intoxication on the blood pressure in the rat. *Amer J Med Sci, 258:*359–365, 1969.

69. Iverson, L. L., Glowinski, J., and Axelrod, J.: The physiological disposition and metabolism of norepinephrine in immunosympathectomized animals. *J Pharmacol Exp Ther, 151:*273–284, 1966.

70. Bornschein, R. L., Michaelson, I. A., and Fox, D.: Lead exposure in lactating rodents: a dose response determination of lead in maternal blood and milk and neonatal blood and brain. *Pharmacol, 17:*212, 1975.

71. Hejtmancik, M. R., Jr., Dawson, E. B., and Williams, B. J.: Tissue distribution of lead in pups nourished by lead-poisoned mothers. *Fed Proceed, 36:*405, 1977.

72. William, B. J., Griffith, W. H., Albrecht, C. M., Pirch, J. H., and Hejtmancik, M. R., Jr.: Effect of chronic lead treatment on some cardiovascular responses to norepinephrine in the rat. *Toxicol Appl Pharmacol, 40:*407–413, 1977.

73. Hejtmancik, M. R., Jr., and Williams, B. J.: Lead exposure and norepinephrine cardiotoxicity: participation of the vagus nerve. *Pharmacol, 19:*134, 1977.

74. Hejtmancik, M. R., Jr. and Williams, B. J.: Effects of chronic lead exposure on the direct and indirect components of the cardiac response to norepinephrine. *Toxicol Appl Pharmacol, 51:*239–245, 1979.

75. Hejtmancik, M. R., Jr., and Williams, B. J.: Time and level of perinatal lead exposure for the development of norepinephrine cardiotoxicity. *Res Comm Chem Pathol Pharmacol, 24:*367–375, 1979.

76. Goldman, D., Hejtmancik, M. R., Jr., Williams, B. J., and Ziegler, M. G.: Noradrenergic effects of lead in the rat. *Pharmacol, 20:*186, 1978.

77. Williams, B. J., Griffith, W. H., Albrecht, C. M., Pirch, J. H., Hejtmancik, M. R., Jr., and Nechay, B. R.: Cardiac effects of lead poisoning. In Brown, S. S. (Ed.): *Clinical Chemistry and Toxicology of Metals.* Oxford, Elsevier-North Holland Biomed. Press, 1977, pp. 127–130.

Chapter 5

IMMUNOTOXICOLOGY AND CHEMICAL CARCINOGENESIS

Joseph K. Prince

ABSTRACT

The influence of environmental chemicals on mammalian systems has been given much attention over the last several years. Bioassays of a chronic duration as well as short-term genetic assays have been developed with an eye toward the early recognition of the occurrence of a lesion in some target organ. Physiological and biochemical changes are targeted for analysis and surveillance in an effort to develop a screen that will signal the possibility of the occurrence of chronic disease.

Although the liver and kidney have been most intensively investigated, other systems have been used in this effort to establish an early warning system. The majority of the studies carried out have not taken into account the possibility that the immune system may be the ideal vehicle for such bioassays. For whatever reasons, investigators have underestimated the importance of the immune system as

The author wishes to acknowledge helpful comments and suggestions contributed to the author by Dr. M. M. Yokoyama, M.D., Ph.D., Director of Clinical Immunology, and Dr. John Bederka Ph.D., Chief of Toxicology and Pharmacometrics, of the University of Illinois Hospital and Medical School Staff.

The author also wishes to acknowledge the very helpful clerical assistance provided by Mrs. Debbie Fript, who did the typing and editing of the manuscript.

The author also accepts the blame for any errors or inconsistencies which may be found, and requests any reader to please notify the author of such mistakes as may occur, without intent.

related to disease states. This author feels that a nucleus of information has been developed by immunological investigators to indicate that the immune system organs and tissue (thymus, spleen, bone marrow, lymphocytes, monocytes) may provide a fertile soil for such investigations that attempt to provide early detection of capacity for chronic disease by environmental chemicals.

Immune deficiency or modulation of the immune response has been known for many years. Irradiation, malnutrition, thymectomy and certain anticancer drugs currently in use are proven to cause a change in the immune system. Although the immune system is complex and not completely understood, sufficient information is available to indicate that various elements in the immune system appear quite sensitive to chemicals.

It is well established that active cells are the most sensitive to chemicals. A good deal of information has been developed on the use of anticancer agents and their capability to induce secondary and tertiary cancers in patients undergoing anticancer treatment. Some of the changes associated with such treatment at the cellular level are also seen *in vivo* and *in vitro* and of course raises the question of whether this activity can be at work during exposure to environmental chemicals? This author feels that there are some relationships that make the next decade in immunotoxicological research possibly the most exciting and potentially the most important.

Introduction

During the last five years, many of us have heard the statement that "a large number of cancers may have their etiology in the environment." This statement helped to propel an already energetic national desire to seek cancer causes and cures. Although there are many different opinions as to the actual numbers of cancer cases contributed by the various environmental factors, it has been generally agreed upon, among biomedically oriented research scientists, that environmental carcinogenesis is a real entity.[1] In an effort to seek a cure or to begin a prevention program, the environmental chemicals that present a carcinogenic risk to humans, are an ideal target for investigation.[2]

In order to establish some measure of risk, predictive toxicology has had to use the various available tools; epidemiology, statistical extrapolations of pharmacological dose response studies, the multiple specie end target organ bioassays, microbial, biochemical studies, and chemical structure relationships.[4-9] These tools, used cautiously, have served us very well. However, the fact that human data is lacking in a majority of the cases has been a source of consternation.

Recent developments in the area of immunology have provided a nucleus of data and of concepts that may help resolve some of these problems associated with extrapolations to humans. Although immune mechanisms and the system has not been defined absolutely, research data has been developed that shows that immune system cells (small lymphocytes, T and B cells, macrophages) and products such as lymphokines play a very important role in the body's immune reaction to possible pathology from microbial infection, graft rejection, and tumour production.

The fact that these cells are readily accessible and are human tissue present in extensive amounts in peripheral blood and have potential for rapid proliferation makes them an ideal vehicle for the study of potential toxicity.

Predictive Toxicology in Retrospect

Epidemiology is the discipline that integrates the impact of the various determinants involved in the disease process. In assessing environmental hazards, it has been used as a tool that helps to provide direction toward actual laboratory investigations. The statistical correlations of the distribution of the determinants of disease have been able to relate the possible chemical toxicants capable of causing pathology to the occasion of disease states among humans who have been exposed. Thus, epidemiology has been an important tool in providing the first step in the process of predictive toxicology—helping to determine in many cases whether a suspect chemical warrants investigation.[3,11,12,13]

Microbial assays have supported predictive toxicology due to the successes of Ames and McCann in establishing aberrations seen in mutagenesis assays as being related to the process of carcinogenesis.[14,15,16] The philosophical basis for this procedure lay in the fact that a chemical capable of causing DNA related lesions could be detected in microbial systems. If a chemical had the capacity to cause mutations in microbial cells, then genetic toxicity was a reality. Using the strain of *Salmonella typhimurium*, which has a histidine negative mutation, Ames and co-workers were able to show that exposure to chemicals causing genetic lesions did cause a reversion or back mutation. The normal Salmonella cell was modified by introducing membrane defects so a chemical could enter. The excision repair system had to be neutralized so that any lesion that could occur remained, and a bacterial plasmid was introduced to insure errors in DNA replication. Finally, rat liver extract was introduced to provide a mammalian metabolic system for activation of the chemical that may not be a direct carcinogen and requires transformation.

Since this system was introduced, others[17,18] have validated the assay system using hundreds of chemicals and have reported that approximately 90 percent of the chemicals tested, which were reported in animal systems to be carcinogenic, were in fact mutagenic in the Ames assay system. Although the correlation is fairly good, caution and prudence must be exercised. Doctor U. Saffiotti of the National Cancer Institute has expressed confidence in the Ames system as having the ability to predict carcinogenic potential, but also added that animal bioassays, using mammalian species are required as conclusive evidence of a chemicals' ability to cause carcinogenesis.[19]

When an appropriate experimental design is used, the mammalian bioassay generates the biological data that has been most sensitive in determining whether a given chemical may have carcinogenic potential. Due to the fact that animals used for carcinogenesis bioassays are highly inbred, some strains may express a predisposing genetic tendency toward the occurrence of neoplastic response from chemical exposures. It was therefore recommended by the National Academy of Sciences[21] that carcinogenic studies be carried out in multiple species of mammalian laboratory animals, so that any expression of a genetic lesion causing neoplastic response be validated or supported as much as possible. Animals, as do humans, have varying susceptibilities, so that the larger data base presents a greater possibility of providing effective extrapolation when predicting possible toxicity.

Anderson and Schein[23] have used the dog and monkey to provide a suitable overlap in combined studies on anticancer chemotherapeutics and found that they were in fact very favorable predictors in preclinical studies. However, the size and cost of such large animals for carcinogenesis assay, given the large number of chemicals in the environment, would present an extreme cost burden in dollars and in human resources.

Carcinogenic or teratological studies have been reported using many species.[24,25] Clegg[26] has indicated that the mouse has provided the most success, but he and Jensen[27] caution that this specificity alone is unsuitable for establishing carcinogenic response. Organ tissue morphology is different; rate of onset of polyploidy, biochemical-enzymic differences, and rough to smooth endoplasmic reticulum change during exposure cause a great deal of difficulty in interpretation of the actual pathology. They do suggest however, such data should be used as a warning signal for further study.

In their report on principals for evaluating environmental chemicals, the National Academy of Sciences (NAS)[21] recommends the use of randomly bred hamster, rat, and mouse as the animal species ideal for carcinogen bioassay.[20] Once again, this is no guarantee of successfully being able to predict human toxicity, but it is all that we have developed up to the present time.

Similar arguments exist for any of the animal species that are used in carcinogenic bioassay. The everpresent reality is that thus far the multiple species bioassay data have provided the best evidence for extrapolating possible chronic pathology from exposure to environmental chemicals.

The recent megamouse study reported by Littlefield et al.[28] has confirmed that the dose-response studies performed on some 26,000 plus mice has validated that such information is absolutely necessary, from a standpoint of both dose and time. He has reported that given different lengths of time of exposure to 2-acetylaminofluorene, an animal could respond with two different end points. Mice that were dosed for eighteen months and sacrificed later showed urinary bladder neoplasms; they also required continual presence of the carcinogen although the neoplastic response was induced early in the study. However, in animals that were exposed for thirty-three months, doing serial sacrifices, a liver neoplasm became evident only late in the study, although it was induced early during exposure and did not require the continual presence of the carcinogen.

This data provides substantial evidence of the necessity of the long-term bioassay. A product of that study was a confirmation of a principle applied to regulatory function in public health programs that "there is no level of exposure greater than zero for a toxic substance, which can be assumed to be without harmful effect."[28]

In contrast to that principal, risk benefit analyses have been introduced based on the public's right of acceptability of possible adverse effect to a given chemical exposure. The calculated risk allows some level of a toxin to coexist in the realm of human existence, correlated with the fact that humanity derives some benefit from that coexistence. In order to calculate that "level of acceptability," it is necessary to extrapolate from the dose of the experiment, associating some end point with a given level and length of time of the exposure. A source of consternation has been, which part of the curve to use when calculating allowable dose to exposed humans.[29-35] Based on the data of the megamouse study, both lesions are induced, in their respective tissues, early in the exposure, suggesting a linear no threshold dose-response. Thus the lower end of the dose curve would be the ideal place to begin extrapolations.[28] Although this philosophy is not espoused by all, it is a practical approach that can provide consistency, assuming the data from bioassays provide sufficient evidence that chronic pathology is a real possibility. Wilson,[36] with some reservations, supports this philosophy, suggesting it is useful for making comparisons with benefits easier to calculate.

The point I have tried to make is that regardless of the method(s) being utilized, problems exist that prevent the unanimous acceptance of any of the given assay systems. Even when taken in concert, the major stumbling block has been that, we do not have information as to how this material will react in humans.

Cellular Basis of Toxicology

The influence of environmental chemicals on the various bio-chemical, morphological, and histopathological parameters has been intensively investigated in various laboratory animals. Epidemiological and statistical analyses have produced more sophisticated and complex mathematical formulas dealing with the extrapolation of dose-response levels and the prediction of toxic associations. Since our predictive ability and the skill we use in evaluating exposure are dependent upon basic biological processes, it is important and prudent that we should direct our energies to answer the basic questions describing how toxicity occurs at the cellular level. Disturbances at the membrane, cytoplasmic, or nuclear levels and at micromolecular structure-activity levels need to be very carefully analyzed to determine the sites and modes of toxicity. Whether for acute or chronic toxicity, these are the fundamental questions that must be answered in order to determine the levels of chemicals humans may tolerate without adverse effect. This is not a new or reorganized philosophy, but a reconfirmation of the original principles laid down by our toxicological forefathers.

As the numbers of chemicals entering into the environment have increased, the long-term bioassays for all chemicals becomes less and less possible due to the length of time and large costs involved. Sequentially, it becomes more important to further develop cellular bioassays as genetic defect predictors. The quicker response time and reduced costs are obvious benefits, although extrapolation is a difficult constraint. Since the correlation of animal responses to human situations are problematical, I suggest we devote more of our attention and energies toward use of human cells. Since the protection and well being of human life is our ultimate end point, data that can be derived from culture and analysis of human cells can provide us with the best evidence for making predictions and risk assessments.

Immune Cell Analyses

One area that has not been well investigated but deserves attention is the human immune system. Vos[10] as well as Silkworth and Loose,[37] have found evidence that supports the concept that environmental chemicals can produce modifications in the activities of the immune system cells. Antibody mediated resistance, cell mediated resistance, as well as increased levels of mortality due to lowered resistance to bacterial infections have been reported in their reviews. Silkworth proposes that cellular and humoral mediated responses may be the appropriate indicators of environmental toxicity. He indicates they are quite sensitive, they can be conveniently evaluated, and he has had limited success using this test system in the evaluation of polychlorinated biphenyls (PCBs), Arochlor 1016 (ACLR), and hexachlorobenzene (HCB). Taylor[38] has analyzed various immune functions in the guinea pig during dietary studies; however, he had conflicting results due to various other factors that could not be controlled. Luster et al.,[39] as well as Luster and Faith,[40] have evaluated the rationale for using immunocompetence as a form of laboratory investigations. They recommend using multiple parameters of study to properly evaluate environmental chemical effects, since normal immune responses are dependent upon macrophages and at least three sets of lymphocytes. These cells interact among themselves and with various cell products (lymphokines and/or complement), so it can become quite complicated. However, the studies they performed did show that exposure to various chemicals produced immune-cell modulation. Dean et al.[41] have examined cell and humoral mediated immunocompetence and also recommend multiple parameter assays, with most of them dealing with systems designed to study tumour/cancer.[10,37–41]

It is obvious that since the immune system deals with a large population of cells of human origin that are available from the peripheral blood, it is an ideal group of cells in which to study toxicity.

Since these cells are present in the circulating peripheral blood, we can correlate their reactions to chemical exposure in a realistic manner, because it is similar to an environmental exposure. Chemicals that are taken in by humans must be absorbed and transported through the circulating blood, which provides the media for close association and residence time. Generally speaking, most chemicals are not biotransformed within the absorptive area of the intestinal tract. In their contact with the blood elements during circulation, not only do you get contact, but also a realistic mode of how and/or what may occur given a chemical and a sensitive or susceptible cell. Cellular response may be at the membrane surface, within the cytoplasmic confines, at the genetic-nuclear level or at all levels. Since immune lymphocytes can be stimulated into differentiation, they can show sensitivity at all levels, making them an ideal vehicle to study cell toxicity modes. With that type of information, immuno– and predictive-toxicology would greatly benefit.

Since immunotoxicology is at its infancy, large amounts of input in developing additional methodologies for detecting cellular determinants and/or receptors and for characterizing pathways and/or molecular constituents are needed. It is a complex task, but these areas must be explored and the quantification of such reactions at the cell level must be identified if we are to gain any further skill in prediction and extrapolating doses to humans.

Immunotoxicology: The Link to Humans?

The immune defense is a dual system composed of natural nonspecific barriers such as skin keratin and pH, of the natural mucociliary barriers as well as the normal bacterial flora that act to prevent bacteria from penetrating. A third nonspecific mechanism begins operating when that first barrier has been breached. Macrophages and polymorphonuclear leucocytes, together with specific humoral soluble factors and lymphokines, act in concert to sequester, degrade, and neutralize the material recognized as foreign.

If these natural and nonspecific barriers have been overwhelmed, the second and more specific defense mechanism comes into play. It involves the activation of lymphocytes that are preprogrammed to combat infection. These lymphocytes are the main element of this system and compose the basis of the humoral and cell mediated immune defense mechanisms. They are indistinguishable morphologically, but, because of differences in the programming sequences, the lymphocytes have different capabilities.

Totipotent (or pluripotent) stem cells derived from the bone marrow are distributed to the peripheral circulation and home in on certain tissue for education and processing. Lymphocyte clones are processed by the thymus gland and are programmed with certain specific surface antigens and cellular memory for use in response to fungi, parasites, intracellular viral infections, tissue grafts and cancer cells. These are the T-lymphocytes, and are responsible for cellular mediated response. That is the response whereby the T-cell is mobilized or stimulated to seek out the foreign material for specific reaction and neutralization. Another group of lymphocytes are processed by gut associated lymphoid tissue (GALT), the supposed equivalent of bursa tissue in the avian models and are then called B-cells. They respond to bacterial infection by transformation into a plasma cell that secretes antibodies. The antibodies are located in the peripheral blood, circulating about until they meet an antigen and then begin the process of neutralization and digestion. Each lymphocyte (T or B) has received specific information during processing and is a clone with a response specificity. The specificity is due to chemical markers imbedded in cell surface conformations that are sensitive only to specific antigens. There are some populations of lymphocytes that although thought to be end cells, have been shown to live for many years and can recirculate from lymph node to lymph and to blood.[42]

Another lymphocyte population that does not possess either immunoglubulin (B) or T-cell surface markers is present and they are called null cells. They are considered to be involved in target cell killing termed *antibody dependent cell mediated cytotoxicity* (AD CC).*

Genetic Regulation

Immune responses are controlled genetically by a series of linked genes known in mice as the major histocompatibility complex (MHC) and in humans as the HLA complex. A similar series of genes has been identified in each mammalian species examined. This phenomena was discovered when guinea pigs inoculated with an antigenic complex of Dinitrophenyl conjugated poly l-lysine (PLL) responded by demonstrating antibody production and delayed hypersensitivity. Strain #2 responded well; however, strain #13 responded poorly. This was taken as evidence that the

---

*The reader is urged to consult one of the currently available texts on immunology for more detailed information.

specific response is due to the carrier, poly l-lysine, and its specific relationship to the PLL gene, which has the capacity to respond.[45]

Further studies were carried out using variations of polymers of amino acids, and seperate genes have been delineated. Strain #2 responded to a copolymer of glutamic acid and alanine (random grouping of AA's) but no response was seen in strain #13. On the other hand, strain #13 responded well to glutamic acid and tyrosine, but strain #2 did not. F1 generation hybrids (13 × 2) however responded to both immunogens, indicating that two different genes were involved, with both having the gene indicating a capacity to respond.

Further observations demonstrated that the ability to respond was linked to the MHC locus. Since that development, genetic control of immune responses and of antigens evoking allograft recognition have been localized to the H–2 gene complex of mouse chromosome #17, and the human leukocyte antigen (HLA) complex in the human on chromosome #6. In the mouse, two regions have been identified: H–2k and H–2d, which determine tissue transplantation antigens and cellular immune cytotoxicity, and the "I" region, which controls induction of immune responses. The H–2k and H–2d regions have been shown to code for the cell *surface antigens* that serve as targets for cell mediated immune reactions as well as the antibody response. This mechanism, which identifies some surface factor of the cell, is used not only to recognize allograft differences, but also plays a role in the recognition of an individual's own cells, which may become changed or altered as in viral infection or neoplastic disease. The mixed lymphocyte reaction is controlled by these loci, and they will proliferate and take up radio thymidine if cells from two different individuals are mixed together. If the cells come from individuals with identical MHC loci, there will be no reaction, and no thymidine will be incorporated. Thus, such an activity as normal response to nonself invasion could be upset should a given gene be affected by a chemical exposure. Since the cell's surface markers and determinants are expressions of genetic activity, those surface membranes may have unusual conformations that could be identified.

Immuneosurveillance

Cell Surface Recognition System

Within the immune defense system there exists a mechanism that has the capacity to recognize the foreign nature of intrusions into a host. Bacterial infections occur, and the antibody response causes neutralization. Foreign tissue graft (allograft) causes the cell mediated response to reject that tissue. Particulate material is sequestered, and phagocytosis causes the degradation of such material till it becomes an innocuous residual body or is discharged from the host. In each case, the immune system recognizes that this material is not identified as self, and sets about to remove the invasion. The immune system has developed and matured in each host, whereby it has learned to recognize the tissue it was associated with during its process of maturation and development. It can distinguish between self and nonself.

The T-lymphocytes, responsible for cell mediated immunity, are part of the internal policing system that is supposed to recognize aberrant cells and remove them from the system. It is able to recognize these cells by surface determinants that reflect the aberrant nature of the cell and would not be found on a normal cell.[43] It is this change in surface antigen markers that separates the self from nonself recognition scheme. This concept was developed for experimental studies in which "nude" (athymic) mice lack the ability to reject tissue grafts because of the defect in the processing of lymphocytes into T-cells.[44] Thus, the animal cannot respond to the foreign nature of a transplanted tumour cell and provides an acceptable medium for growth of various tumour cells, whereas, if a tumour is transplanted into a normal mouse, there is a rejection of the tumour tissue. It is now generally accepted that most transplanted tumours have tumour specific antigens that are the basis for the induction of the immune rejection reaction. They are called tumour specific transplantation antigens (TSTA's).

This concept of tumour specific antigens has had a profound impact on tumour immunology. Mice that were inoculated with polyoma virus were later capable of rejecting a polyoma tumour that was grafted onto a synegenic mouse (genetically identical). This was interpreted as an example of the immune system's recognition that the tumour tissue was indeed foreign and that preimmunization was directed at these surface markers. It was also hypothesized that the immune system was capable of limiting tumour development. A logical extension of that concept held that if there is a condition that exists in the animal that modifies or alters the immune system's capabilities to respond to a nonself entity (immunemodulation), then the variant cell or foreign entity can take hold, develop and mature into perhaps a disease state.[42-45]

Immune Modulation

Immune modulation can take variable forms of stimulation or suppression, and it can be specific or general. Stimulation (specific) of the system *directly* occurs in immunization with microbial cells or products or *indirectly* as in passive transfer of serum, cells, or cell products among histocompatible donors and recipients. There are also nonspecific or general responses that can occur as with *Bacillus calmette guerin* (BCG), *Corynebacterium parvum*, levamisole, and pokeweed. These cells or products are referred to as mitogenic since they are nonspecific and have the ability to stimulate B and T cells, as well as macrophages or the complement system.

Immunosuppression, on the other hand, is the reduction of available immune elements directly or indirectly. Lymphoid drainage, cytoxic drugs, antilymphocyte serum are direct, as is thymectomy, which will reduce T-cell populations and response. Irradiation is general suppression of the immune response. Bursectomy in fowl will lead to loss of B-cell response. Indirectly, one can also modify the response by increasing or reducing the levels of corticosteroids or using various known antiinflammatory agents.

Based on this ability to modify the immune response, medical science began the use of chemotherapeutics. In the clinical sense, the goal is to suppress or eliminate the ability to produce an immune response to specific antigen while allowing other antigens to evoke a response, as in organ transplants.[45,46] Such suppression has been used in the clinical treatment of neoplastic disease. Some cancer cells, as do bone marrow cells and intestinal mucosa, show an extremely rapid growth rate and, additionally, may have an abnormal complement of nucleic acids. Alkylating agents as well as blocking agents are used to interfere with metabolism of such cells. Because some neoplastic cells metabolize at accelerated rates, they are more likely to pick up higher doses of antimetabolic agents. However, the immune lymphoid system cells are also more active so they can also be affected to a greater degree. Induction of an immunocompromised individual through the use of chemicals has become well known in cases of clinical chemotherapy.[46]

Immune Deficiency and Malignancy

One of the most significant advances in cancer information is the finding that immunodeficient states are associated with an increased incidence of malignancy. Kersey[81] has shown that patients who have naturally occurring states of immunodeficiency such as Wiskott-Aldrich disease, Ataxia telangiectasia, or agammaglobulinemia have an unusually high incidence of malignant disease.

Numerous experimental bioassays are cited in his review, showing that immune suppression facilitates transplants of malignant cells, increases a normally low incidence of viral or chemically induced cancers and accelerates growth of metastases.

Immunosuppressive therapy has been used for some twenty odd years and has had a significant impact in producing secondary and tertiary cancers in patients who were under such treatment. Penn[46] has been maintaining a tumour registry of patients who were on immunosuppressive therapy and classified them into five groups with the following results.

Patients with Transplanted Cancers

Sixty-one patients who had received organ transplants from donors who were neoplastic or within several months subsequent to donation developed evidence of malignancy showed that twenty-one patients or 34 percent had evidence of transmitted cancers. Cessation of immunosuppressive therapy and removal of the graft resulted in the complete disappearance of the disseminated neoplasms.

Transplant Patients with De-novo Malignancies

In a long-term follow up of the University of Colorado series of renal homografts, 32 of 564 patients developed cancer, an incidence of 5.7 percent. The Denver Transplant Tumor Registry has data on 401 *de novo* cancers that have occurred in 378 patients who have received kidneys. The average age of the patients were thirty-nine years old (range eight to seventy years) and the neoplasms occurred from one month to one hundred fifty four months (1 to 154) after the transplant (average 32 months). After the transplants, the following immunosuppressive procedures were used: Prednisone, Azothioprine, anti-lymphocyte globulin (ALG), Actinomycin, cyclophosphomide. Radiation, splenectomy, thymectomy and thoracic duct fistula procedures were also in use. In conjunction with ALG treatment, 6-mercaptopurine, methotrexate, and azaserine were also used.

The patients receiving irradiation, splenectomy, thymectomy, or thoracic duct drainage treatment accounted for 217 *de novo* cancers, while the patients on pharmacologic therapy accounted for the remaining 164 cancers. The development of malignancy could not be related to the use of any one agent, but appeared to be an effect of the general immunosuppression. A significant finding was that the incidence rate of solid lymphomas among the organ transplant patients was disproportionally higher than the general population. One variety, Reticulum Cell Sarcoma, was calculated to be 350 times more common. The lymphoma patients were slightly younger than the other cancer patients (36.5 versus 40 years old), and the tumours appeared earlier than the other cancer patients (twenty-three versus thirty-five months). The solid lymphomas occurred in ninety-five patients with the following breakdown:

Reticulum cell sarcomas 68
   (One patient also had a Kaposi's sarcoma.)
Kaposi's sarcoma 11
Lymphoma 8
   (Including 1 plasma cell lymphoma).
Lymphosarcoma 5
Lymphoreticular malignancy 2
Hodgkins Disease 1
Histiocytic Reticulosis (?) 1

Non Transplant Patients Treated with Immunosuppressives (Antiinflammatory therapy)

Data has been collected that indicates that of seventy patients who have been under antiinflammatory therapy, seventy-two cancers developed during treatment with various agents.

Disease	No. Cases	Therapy	No. Cases	Cancer Type	No. Cases
Psoriasis	24	Methotrexate	23	Lymphoma	4
		Aminopterin	3	Leukemia	1
		Other	8	Skin	5
				Misc.	16
Renal Disease	13	Azathioprine	7	Skin	5
		Cyclophosphamide	7	Lymphoma	2
		Other	10	Misc.	6
Rheumatoid Arthritis	10	Cyclophosphamide	8	Lymphoma	5
		Other	8	Leukemia	3
				Lymphoma	2
				Misc.	4
Systemic Lupus Erythematosus	7	Cyclophosphamide	3	Kaposi's Sarcoma	1
		Azotheoprine	6		
		Other	6		
Other Inflamatory Diseases	16	Agents Used (as above, alone or as combined)	31	Cancers (Lymphomas, Leukemias, Hodgkins, and cancer of skin, bladder, colon, bronchus.)	16

Neoplastic Diseased Patients Without Transplants

In nontransplant patients with neoplasms receiving immunosuppressive cancer therapy, Penn[46] and Kersey[81] showed that second and even third tumours have arisen during treatment with chemotherapeutics. Of 185 patients with tumours treated with either Melphalan, cyclophosphamide, busulfan, 6-mercaptopurine, chlornaphazine, chlorambucil, thiotepa, methotrexate, and prednisone, alone or in combination, 194 new malignancies developed. Various leukemias accounted for eighty-two of the new malignancies: thirty-five lymphomas, twenty bladder carcinomas, two cases of cancer of the cervix, and one Hodgkins disease occurred. The remainder of the cases were various and miscellaneous forms of malignancy and totalled fifty-five.

Acute leukemia occurred in thirty-nine cases where the patients originally had multiple myeloma. Twenty-seven solid lymphomas developed in cases where the patient's original neoplasm was chronic granulocytic leukemia. These unusual occurrences would tend to dispel any ideas that these cancers were transition forms of the existing malignancy. Thus, one can cautiously extrapolate the data and identify a significant association between the development of malignancy of lymphoid elements and the use of chemicals that have the capability of suppressing elements in the immunc/host defense system. (Chlornaphazine is the one agent capable of directly causing cancer in man since it metabolizes to betanaphthylamine. It has caused bladder cancer in aniline dye workers.)

Leukemias and Chemical Immune Modulation

Of the four major types of cytological leukemia, myeloid and lymphatic constitute the greatest percentage. Myeloid cases peak out at about 60 percent of all leukemias at age thirty to forty, then declines thereafter. The lymphatic type has the highest prevalence in children peaking at about 50 percent and then declines till age thirty to forty. It then rises to 60 percent peak between ages eighty to ninety. On the way up to its peak, the lymphatic type passes myeloid type leukemia at about seventy years of age.[47]

An epidemiological study of solvent exposure and leukemia was conducted among rubber workers by McMichael et al.[48] indicating that an association between leukemia and jobs that involved using solvents existed. Prior to this time, Kessler and Lillienfeld (1969) as well as Vigliani and Saita[49] had prepared papers indicating they thought that the current evidence supported benzene, phenylbutazone, and chloramphenicol as being luekemogens; however, they had found little epidemiological evidence to support this posture. McMichael et al.[48] had analyzed some 6600 co-workers (male rubber workers) who were working during the years 1964 to 1972, but had an employment duration of twenty-five years. They were followed for nine years with a 1 percent loss. Matched controls were also analyzed, with standard mortality ratios and proportional mortality ratios calculated. Of the various relationships that were analyzed, the association of death from lymphatic leukemia with a history of having worked in solvent exposure environment stood out. It is of interest that the lymphatic leukemia stands out as associated with solvent exposure jobs. This leukemia tends to be the myeloblasic or the stem cell type. McMichael had indicated that the leukemogenic effects may have been the result of concomitant exposure to other solvents that were used in the rubber industry.

However, Infante et al.[50] studied a population of workers who were occupationally exposed to only benzene during 1940 to 1949 and who were followed until 1975. Comparisons with two control groups show a significant excess of observed leukemia (p less than 0.002). A five fold excess risk of all leukemias and a ten fold excess risk of death from myeloid and monocytic leukemias combined were demonstrated in the comparison between populations. The environments of those workers were analyzed, and records have shown that the benzene levels were generally lower than the recommended limits at the time they were measured.

The observations are in agreement with Vigliani and Saita,[49] whereby a specific type of leukemia is associated with the exposure to benzene. The myelogenous or monocytic leukemia has been shown to correlate very well with the exposure and confirms the suspicion that benzene is a powerful bone marrow poison.[53] Goldstein[51] has written an excellent review of the toxic hemopoeitic effects of benzene exposure. These effects, although somewhat complicated by concomitant exposure in some cases, are fairly well demonstrated.

The mechanism by which this toxicity occurs is not known; however, the alteration of *stem cell* function is apparent.[51,52,53] Occupationally exposed persons as well as laboratory animal studies have shown chromosomal abnormalities, and correlates well with the known clinical picture of benzene toxicity.[54,55,56] Goldstein has reported that in mice chronically exposed to 100 ppm of benzene, leukopenia, due primarily to lymphocytopenia, was clearly demonstrated. These manifestations of pancytopenia may represent a destruction of the stem cells, failure of the cells to mature, or prevention of differentiation at some critical stage. Other agents known to produce pancytopenia act in this fashion through modification of nuclear material. They include ionizing radiation chloromycetin, vinblastine, mitomycin, puromycin, colchicine and cytochalasin B. Many of these latter compounds have been used in clinical treatment of malignancy.

Forni et al.[52] carried out cytogenic studies and have confirmed chromosomal aberrations occurring in peripheral blood lymphocytes, due to benzene exposure.

If one examines the ontogeny of lymphocytes, it is readily apparent that bone marrow stem cells develop into two different lines of cells. The one line produces hemopoietic precursors, and the second line produces the lymphoid cells. Logically, interference at the stem cell level is bound to affect both the blood elements as well as the immune system elements. Laboratory investigations have observed pancytopenias such as monocytic, and myelogenous leukemias due to benzene exposure also show stem cells that have produced abnormal mature erythrocytes, which further supports stem cell nuclear function interference.

Wolman[54] has indicated that ample evidence is present to show that chromosomal aberrations can be induced through exposure to benzene. Gaps and junction breaks have been observed in cultured human cells (leukocytes and HeLa cells) at 1.1 or 2.2×10^{-3} M. benzene. Higher doses caused inhibited DNA synthesis. Peripheral lymphocytes stimulated by phytohemaglutinin (PHA) exposed to benzene for seventy-two hours revealed both numerical and structural alterations. Aneuploidy and chromosome breakage occurred seven and eight times more frequently in treated cells.

Immunochemicals and Cancer

Advances in pharmacological therapy has produced problems as well as remissions in the treatment of disease states. Patients who have been treated with antihypertensive, antiarrythmic agents as well as antubercular or anticonvulsive agents have shown to be susceptible to a syndrome related to the immune disease called systemic lupus erythematosus (SLE).[42,44,45] In SLE, the patient develops antibodies stimulated by the patient's own cellular material, especially the nuclear elements. It affects various tissues, and has a fatal form. One of the major findings in diagnosis has been the presence of an LE cell (polymorphonuclear leucocyte— PMN) that contains phagocytized nuclear material. This cell is formed as a consequence of reaction between an antibody present that can bind cellular nucleoproteins. Presumably the mechanism involves the lymphocytic nuclei that reacts with the antibody. Lymphocytes become saturated on their active sites, and PMN cells come to engulf the swollen lymphocytes. Digesting away (phagocytosis) the remainder of the lymphocyte, the PMN packages the nucleoprotein material as a residual body called LE. Although this disease is usually virally induced, therapeutic agents such as diphenylhydantoin, isoniazid, hydralazine, and procainamide have induced the syndrome that generally disappears upon withdrawal of the drug. These mechanisms that induce the SLE syndrome are not yet well understood; however, chemical influence on the immune system has produced antibodies that include anti-DNA, antinucleoprotein, antihistones, antinucleolar RNA, and antibodies to fibrous or particulate nucleoproteins. The importance of these data reflect that exogenous chemicals, which modify or influence biological systems, have unusual effects that are not always readily apparent. How this important defense mechanism has been modulated by interplay with chemicals is unknown, but any real capacity to effect nuclear material creates greater possibilities of biological dysfunction.

Zarrabi et al.[57] studied four groups of humans under treatment for some two and one-half years, with chlorpromazine and various other antipsychotic drugs. The main observation was the prevalence of immunologic and thromboplastic coagulative disorders. In patients on long-term chlorpromazine, the authors found that patients had increased levels of serum IgM, 405 ± 55 (in chlorpromazine treated patients), whereas controls had 157 ± 23, and normal is considered to range from 60 to 250: patients who were given combined therapy, chlorpromazine plus another drug, for the same length of time showed levels of serum IgM at 493 ± 75. Other antipsychotics used were thioridizine, trifluoperazine, thiothixene, perphenazine, haloperidol, lithium, and amitryptilene. This group alone did not provide any significant differences when comparisons were made between the groups studied. Also noted was an increase in length of partial thromboplastin time. In both instances, significant correlation between increased levels of IgM in serum along with thromboplastin time were noted in relation to dose and duration of therapy. Both groups had a positive antinuclear antibody test (63%), both had nucleoprotein antibodies (58%), and both groups had antibodies to native DNA (40%).

It is interesting to note the authors' conclusion, "the IgM was the coagulation inhibitor," and was identified through immune neutralization and immunoglobulin isolation techniques. A product of the immunological analyses was the finding that the percentage of T-lymphocytes were below normal in thirteen out of forty-one patients treated with Chlorpromazine and twenty out of forty-two patients under single or combined treatment developed splenomegaly.

Recently, Doctor I. Fidler[58] at the Detrich Maryland Cancer Research Center, working with macrophages from mouse peritoneum, found that for some odd reason the macrophages began losing their tumoricidal activity during *in vitro* studies. Ordinarily, such macrophages in the peritoneum are not cytotoxic to tumour cells *in vitro;* however, a lymphokine released by an activated lymphocyte, referred to as macrophage activating factor (MAF) has the ability to stimulate the macrophage to become tumoricidal. Such peritoneal exudate macrophages (PEM) can also be stimulated to become cytotoxic by bacterial products (lipopolysaccharide — LPS), endotoxins, pyran copolymers, double stranded RNA, or during chronic infection with obligate bacteria. The *in vitro* studies were stopped and, in certain cases, the procedure modified because the PEMs were found to have lost the cytotoxic capability. A careful examination of the occurrence of lost activity seemed to correlate with a minor change in the drinking water used for the mouse colonies.

Water fed to the mice had a chlorine level of about twelve to sixteen parts per million (ppm). This high level is necessary to reduce the rate of early death syndrome in the colonies due to *Pseudomonas* infection since the mice had been lethally irradiated.

Due to an unusually high incidence of such early death syndromes, the chlorine level was raised to 25 to 30 ppm, and the experimental studies were carried on as usual.

At the start of the experiment and just before treatment, the mean number of PEMs per mouse was $21 \pm 4 \times 10^6$. One week later the level of PEMs in the mice receiving hyperchlorinated water had decreased to $13 \pm 2 \times 10^6$ per mouse. Controls were yielding $25 \pm 3 \times 10^6$ per mouse. On consecutive weeks, PEM yield increased from the control mice, but mice on hyperchlorinated water had reduced PEMs or remained lower than controls. Mice that were receiving tap water yielded macrophages that when stimulated were tumorcidal *in vitro* to B16 melanoma cells or to UV 112 fibrosarcoma when activated by Concanavalin A-MAF, as measured by release of radioactivity.

The mice drinking hyperchlorinated water exhibited lowered levels of cytotoxic ability for the first two weeks, and, by the end of the third week of treatment, the cells, although stimulated by Con A-MAF, were not tumoricidal.

These studies show that hyperchlorinated water produces profound alterations in the numbers and tumoricidal capacity of PEMs. Lower levels (10-15 ppm) may also exert such influence although over a longer period of time.

Supporting these effects was a report by Fidler that showed that patients on long-term hemodialysis developed acute hemolytic anemia when treated with water that, although filtered by reverse osmosis, has 2 to 4 ppm chlorine. Chlorine compunds brought about a denaturation of the hemoglobin by direct oxidation and also by inhibition of the direct oxidative pathway (Hexose monophosphate shunt) of red blood cells (RBCs). The damage to RBCs was found to be cumulative over several periods of dialysis.

Although the mechanism for this depression of macrophage tumoricidal activity is unknown, Fidler suggests several possibilities. The vacuoles of the macrophage system are probably involved in the cytotoxic mechanism. This has been shown by Hibbs and Weinberg[59] whereby inhibition of the lysosomal enzymes of the macrophages occurs by addition of trypan blue, and stabilization of the lysosomal membranes occurs with the addition of hydrocortisone, and the cytotoxic activity is suppressed.

Macrophages that have been activated by lymphokines have enhanced bactericidal activity, and metabolically are shown to have a four to eight times increase in the uptake of glucose and its oxidation as compared to controls. Since the chlorine (compounds) inhibits the HMPS pathway[59] (that is the major path for glucose oxidation in the RBC's), there is a possibility that chlorine and/or its compounds may sufficiently inhibit glucose oxidation to the point whereby macrophages that have reduced tumouricidal capacity will allow aberrant cells to continue growing and relocalizing! Concurrently, indirect pathology also occurs! Chlorine levels affect erythrocytes' glucose metabolism, and large amounts of hemoglobin degradation products and/or large numbers of damaged RBCs can suppress macrophage tumoridical activity.

Regardless of the mechanism by which the chlorinated water or chlorine compounds may exert their influence, the important fact remains that macrophage activity is compromised. Since it carries a major role in host defense against neoplastic disease, the possibility exists that a host who is exposed to such compounds may in fact become immunocompromised. Silica, carageenan, and trypan blue are substances that also have the ability to suppress macrophages in lab studies have been reported to decrease host resistance against transplantable tumours.

Dandliker et al.[60] recently reported their studies of the effects of pesticides on the immune response. Hamsters (LHC/LAK) five to eight weeks old and weighing about 100 grams were given a dose of pesticide equal to one-half the LD^{50} dissolved in 1 ml of corn oil. Arochlor 1260, Dinoseb, Parathion, pentachloronitrobenzene, piperonyl butoxide, mixed pyrethrins, and resmithrin were administered intragastrically. The animals were examined for an end point of "redness and swelling" (inflammatory response) and change in temperature of the foot pads, as well as histological exam, after an antigenic challenge. Serum antibody titer, binding affinity, and heterogeneity were determined by fluorescent polarization measurements.

The animals were first given an injection of fluorescein labeled ovalbumin, allowed only water *ad lib* for twenty-four hours, and then given a bolus of food with the pesticide by intragastric feeding tube twenty-four hours after the immunization. The most striking feature reported by the authors after immunanalysis indicated marked humoral and cellular immunosuppression to single doses of Dinoseb and Parathion, and a marked stimulation of the cellular response by resmethrin. The other pesticides showed little or no effect under those conditions.

In another study[61] using the pesticides Ametryne, Carbaryl, Chlodimeform, DDT, Malathion, Mirex, and parathion, a single dose of pesticide was given orally at the LD^{50} or the 0.1 LD^{50} five days before, two days before, or two days after immunization with sheep erythrocytes. Assays were then conducted using antibody plaque forming cells four days later. (Plaque forming cells — antibody producing cells that can form a hemolytic plaque in the presence of complement and erythrocytes.) All animals receiving the higher dose exhibited significant depressions in splenic plaque forming cell numbers. Low dose animals receiving the dose for either eight or twenty-eight days prior to immunization exhibited no significant reduction in the antibody plaque forming cell numbers. The author indicates that a lack of information prevents a conclusion as to the efficacy of these compounds on modulating the immune system. Since the methodology only uses one test for the erythrocyte receptor, little can be concluded. This is why multiple parameter assays are necessary.

Faith and Luster[62] have performed extensive investigations on the pre– and postnatal effects of Tetrachlorodibenzodioxin (TCDD) on the immune system and have found that TCDD appears a relatively excellent immunosuppressive in the Fischer/Wistar rat strains. The Fischer strain is reputed to be less of a responder than its Fischer/Wistar cousin. However, dosing of nursing females has shown that the TCDD has the capability of causing immunosuppression in littermates. The effects have lasted as long as 270 days, from three doses to the mother at days zero, seven, and fourteen, applied at five micrograms per kilogram (ug/kg) body weight. At days eighteen and thirty-five, both female and male littermates showed depressed body weight as well as depressed thymic weights. These depressed values were evident at day 128 postdosing. The weight of the spleens were also found to be affected.

Effects of TCDD exposure on the homing patterns of lymphocytes were also studied in these same rat strains. Splenic cells taken from the TCDD exposed rats were injected into nonexposed rats, and the thymus was found to significantly increase the uptake of such cells. Thymic cells taken from nonexposed rats were injected into TCDD exposed rats, and it was found that there was decreased homing ability to the thymus. The authors proposed that a change in cellular metabolism occurred altering the cell membrane, or that insertion of the TCDD into the membrane caused surface alterations, and this change in the cell modified its normal homing patterns. Various investigators have shown such alterations in immune function due to TCDD exposure.[63],[64],[65]

Thigpen[63] has shown that subclinical doses of TCDD had the ability to affect host response, when subsequent exposure to *Salmonella* infection resulted in reduced time to mortality. Thus far, exposure to TCDD has been shown to cause an increase in the susceptibility to bacterial infections (suppression of immune response) as well as suppression of mitogen responsiveness, suppression of the skin graft rejection, and depression of the delayed hypersensitivity response. (Suppression of the T-cell dependent immune functions appears to occur as an isolated response.)

Phenol

Lavia et al.[66] also had occasion to come upon the effects of phenol on immune function through a case of serendipity, as did Fidler. Phenol was being used to disinfect the cages of mice, and was found to be causing depression of the immune response to t-dependent antigens in the time period of four to six weeks. Further analysis of the phenol showed the disinfectant to be a mixture of o-phenylphenol (5.0%), o-benzyl-p-phenol (4.5%), and p-tert-amylphenol (1.0%), OPP, OBP, and PTA, respectively. Such compounds are used in biocides throughout the world.

Oehme[67] has studied the metabolism of one compound, o-phenylphenol (OPP) in the cat and dog and has found that although the two animals metabolize OPP according to two different routes and rates, excessive tissue levels are found in the spleen. Lavia[66] decided to study this phenomena on immune function knowing that the spleen plays a major role in the immune response. Groups of BALB/c female mice were dosed with the phenol derivatives (all three derivatives were used, but each group of mice received only a single compound) at levels of 0.46 milligrams per kilogram (mg/kg) of OPP, 0.41 mg/kg OBP, and 0.09 mg/kg PTA in their drinking water. At weekly intervals, three mice were immunized intraperitoneally with 1.0×10^8 sheep erythrocytes (SRBC). Four days later the number of IgM plague forming cells (PFC) was determined. Before the end of the second week of exposure, 45 percent of the mice showed immunodepressive effects. The response after four weeks showed depression to be occurring in 77 percent of the dosed mice. Comparison of OPP with a mixture of phenol compounds showed the immune depression to be the same, indicating that OPP appears to have the same capacity for immune suppression as the mixture and must be exercising dominance in producing the response. Monocytes (Macrophages) were also analyzed for their capacity to phagocytize yeast cells. This capacity was significantly reduced as compared to controls. Measurement of T and B lymphocyte numbers in control and OPP exposed mice showed no significant differences.

The net effect was that the macrophages appear to have sustained some defect that reduced their ability to present antigen for phagocytosis or may have just resulted in a reduced number of circulating macrophages that could affect the cooperative cell–cell activation upon B-lymphocytes. Archer[68] has also studied the suppression of the immune system using gallic acid, a phenolic derivative, and has concluded that the mouse spleen cells that were studied showed a marked depression of the immune system from such exposure probably at the macrophage level. These data are very important, because it shows that immune suppression has occurred at low dose levels and with short periods of exposure, which situation mimics many of the environmental exposures. This is true especially with drinking water. To extrapolate this evidence without asking other pertinent questions clearly is not yet justified, but when taken in concert with the studies done by others, it can be seen that the immune system is in fact a very sensitive system that may be an ideal vehicle for indicating potential toxicity to humans. Although ultrastructural morphology or DNA damage studies have been used prior to this time for indications of toxicity, it appears that immune cell biochemistry may be more sensitive to such low level doses that are prevalent in the environment and would complement such bioassays.

Metallo Organics

Extensive investigations have been made of the effects of organo tin compounds on the immune system and it has been shown by Seinen and Penninks[69] that Di-n-octyl-tin chloride causes a depletion of lymphocytes in the thymus and thymus dependent areas in the spleen and lymph nodes. There was a dose dependent relationship showing a decrease in the number as well as the viability of thymocytes. Spleen cell numbers and viability were slightly less pronounced, and no effect was found on bone marrow and/or peripheral lymphocytes and/or monocytes. Thymic atrophy reversed upon discontinuation of the exposure. The results of exposure to Di-n-butyl tin chloride was identical to the Di-n-octyl tin chloride. Di-n-ethyl-, and Di-n-propyl tin chloride compounds showed less pronounced effects. In contrast, Di-n-methyl-, Di-n-dodecyl-, and Di-n-octadecyl tin chlorides as well as monooctyl-, tri-n-octyl-, and tetraoctyltinchlorides did not show any thymic atrophy. In this excellent review, they examined a large body of data dealing with lead and cadmium on the immune system and established that the major effect is an increased susceptibility to infection by gram negative bacteria that contain endotoxin. Lead is also shown to decrease the resistance to viral disease, so one can conclude that the humoral response is somehow affected causing B-lymphocyte defects in antibody generation, or perhaps in the modification of circulating antibody molecule itself. Koller,[70] using rabbits dosed with lead acetate, 2200 mg/liter (equal parts per million) in water showed that after ten weeks of exposure, both the primary and secondary response to pseudorabies virus had been depressed. Koller and Kovacic[71] showed that mice dosed with lead acetate had a significantly increased number of IgM plague forming cells to SRBC. This further adds to the complexity of the situation, since the effect may be occurring in the lymphoid organ(s) associated with development of B-cells. Additional cells may be stimulated without proper maturation and/or they may have defective antibody response capability. Chronic low level dosing of lead to rats pre– and postnatally by Faith et al.[72] showed the thymus weights to be suppressed along with decreased responsiveness to

mitogen stimulation of lymphocytes and reduced delayed hypersensitivity response. Of greater importance is the fact that the
offspring of females dosed with 25 or 50 ppm of lead in drinking
water showed no inhibition of growth, as exhibited by body weight
gain, nor overt signs of toxicity. However, the analysis of the
immune system functions of offspring did show decreased mitogen
responsiveness, as well as the depressed delayed hypersensitivity
reaction. The inescapable fact is that some facet of the immune
function has been altered. The doses of 25, 50 ppm lead used for
the mice produced blood levels of 29.3 and 52.8 micrograms per
100 ml blood, which are comparable to blood levels found in
human children, makes currently allowable lead levels somewhat
undesirable. In light of the relationship of humans to lab animals,
and to this evidence, supplied by the more sensitive immunological
indicator, covert toxicity may in fact be occurring[72-74] even at low
levels.

Hoffman and Niyogi[74] have studied metal carcinogens and have
indicated that lead and the other metal salts were able to interfere
with the fidelity of DNA synthesis. Such interference would, if
occurring in the B-cells, have a profound effect on resistance since
the ability to differentiate in lymphocytes is absolutely necessary
for host defense. Should it interfere with the DNA at a small
lymphocyte blast stage perhaps a major clonal species of lymphocyte
could be permanently impaired!

Additional studies by Vos et al.[75] using hexachlorobenzene on
rats has shown the immune system to be stimulated, which con-
trasts other data presented. Sharma[76] has exposed mice to vinyl
chloride and found the immune system lymphocytes to be pro-
foundly stimulated.

Miller[77] and Kagan and Miller[78] also have observed immuno-
stimulation in patients who have asbestosis. Some disturbance
may have occurred in the immune regulatory mechanism, since
they have shown hyperactivity in the humoral immune response,
increased reproduction in the serum globulins, secretory IgA, and
a variety of autoantibodies. The reason for this activity is not
clear; however, asbestos studies done on the lung suggest that
macrophages trying to digest the mineral fibers are damaged,
spilling out lysosomal enzymes, which may bring on autoimmune

pathology. Drath et al.[80] have established that smoke from tobacco causes morphological biochemical and functional alterations in the pulmonary alveolar macrophages, which are functionally impaired with respect to phagocytosis. Since it is well established that macrophages are an integral unit of the immune responses,[79] there is a significant modulation occurring that cannot be denied, but whose total impact is yet to be discovered.

Because of a known role in the immunosurveillance mechanism, the possibility of modulation by environmental chemicals of the immune cells certainly seems an exciting speculation.

Summary

The influence of environmental chemicals upon the public health is of considerable importance. Determining how such chemicals may cause adverse effects upon humans is a continuing problem that perplexes all phases of scientific inquiry. Genetic chronic toxicity and dose responses are defined from animal bioassays and microbial DNA studies for human use, and constitute a major source of controversy among predictive toxicologists.

A major step forward in resolving such problems could be attained with the use of human lymphoid cells, which are readily available from the peripheral circulating blood. The lymphoid cells of the immune system are an integral part of the defense mechanism known as immune surveillance and are very important in the recognition and removal of abberant or malignant cells. It is this relationship that may be disturbed by environmental chemicals and allows carcinogenesis to proceed in susceptible individuals.

The use of immunosuppressive therapy has shown there is an increased frequency of various types of malignant disease associated with continued use of such agents. Secondary as well as tertiary cancers have been produced by therapeutic suppression of the immune system. Concurrently, investigators have also shown that occurrence of malignant disease is also found in individuals with genetic immunodeficiencies at a higher frequency than in immune normal hosts. So it has become apparent that malignant response in a given host may in fact be very seriously dependent upon an immune system that has been somehow compromised.

In vitro and *vivo* studies using pesticides, metallo-organics and various pharmacological agents, have shown that certain activities of lymphoid cells are modulated by the presence of many of these compounds.

Lymphocytes have been either suppressed or stimulated, and either condition may be affecting immune response. The blood monocytes, which play a vital role in the B-cell/T-cell interactions, are shown to be very severely disturbed by excessive amounts of chlorine or hemoglobin degradation products. So, direct or indirect effects can modulate the immune response, showing the sensitivity of the lymphoid population to environmental influence. The cells themselves may become defective through direct action, or the tissue in which they mature and differentiate may be modified, producing an impotent cell.

The cell may be affected at the surface, within the cytoplasm where antigenic determinants are synthesized, or within the nuclear protein and/or chromosomal levels. Thus there exists a cell for all seasons; morphologists, biochemists, immunologists, pure chemists, pure biologists, all will find an abundance of suitable material to investigate. The most rewarding portion of our work may well be that we will be closer to effective extrapolation for human exposure.

Conclusion

The mechanisms whereby chemicals influence the immunological surveillance system are not understood. In fact, there are many who have asked questions that may dull the excitement over the immunosurveillance theory. However, they have not been sufficiently substantiated. What has been elucidated in this presentation is that we cannot deny the influences external chemicals have on the cells and products of tissue from the lymphoid-immune system. The role of chemically induced malignancy in the immune suppressed patients receiving therapy or the excess occurrences of malignant disease in immunodeficient individuals is significant and cannot be ignored. The complexity of the immune system, details of mechanisms, in fact, whether cells or products may be influencing this system is in most cases not known. However, it can be stated that many of the substances mentioned here today are in the environment and they do have immunomodulating effects. How does this role of immunomodulation affect interpretation of previous studies that discerned that a mouse, rat, guinea pig, or some other lab animal has or has not responded with malignancy to a carcinogenic chemical? Have those modulating effects been taken into account in concluding that some chemical is or is not a carcinogen? Clearly such questions can establish a compromised position when making conclusions as to whether any chemical should be allowed in the human environment. Mice, rats, hamsters, and guinea pigs have variable systems. Has the chemical tested caused a depression of the system that allowed some ' virus to induce a cancer? Or has the animal perhaps a depressed immune system, due to repression of genetic expression due to inbreeding that now allows a neoplastic response to occur?

Immunotoxicology is the new kid on the block and is able to ask some very difficult questions. Questions for which we have not all the answers.

In the area of predictive toxicology, however, I would suggest the following. Because immunotoxicology may bring about an additional dimension in extrapolation, I would suggest that future studies be directed toward examining these immune system elements and how they respond to mutagenic or carcinogenic agents. Not only in the lab animal species, but by using the peripheral blood elements from humans. Establishing a tissue culture procedure with human lymphocytes and/or macrophages, even though *in vitro*, would allow function and surface identification studies as well as biochemical investigations to procede and perhaps promote greater confidence when possibly identifying toxic responses to humans. Other human cells have been cultured, such as fibroblasts and the HeLa cells, surely the same could be done for the immune system cells. It would go far in impacting the program of public health for which we are all responsible.

References

1. Kraybill, H. F.: Carcinogenesis induced by trace contaminants in potable water. *Bull New York Acad Medicine, 54:*413, 1978.
2. Smith, J. R.: Government says cancer rate is increasing. *Science, 209:*998, 1980.

3. Doll, Sir Richard: Strategy for detection of cancer hazards to man. *Nature, 265:*589, 1977.

4. Scheiderman, M., and Brown, C. C.: Estimating cancer risks to a population. *Env Health Perspectives, 22:*115, 1978.

5. Rall, David P.: Difficulties in extrapolating the results of toxicity studies in laboratory animals to man. *Environmental research, 2:*360, 1969.

6. Doll, Sir Richard: Epidemiology of cancer: Current perspectives. *Amer Journ of Epidemiology, 4:*396, 1976.

7. Bishop, Yvonne M.: Statistical methods for hazard and health. *Env Health Perspectives, 20:*149, 1977.

8. Lepkowski, Wil: Extrapolation of carcinogenesis data. *Env Health Perspectives, 22:*173, 1978.

9. Rall, David P.: Chemical carcinogenesis and mutagenesis: Introduction to symposium III. Proceedings of the European Society of Toxicology, 1978.

10. Vos, J. G.: Immune suppression as related to toxicology. *CRC Critical Reviews in Toxicology, 5:*67, 1977.

11. Cantor, K. P., and McCabe, L. J.: The epidemiologic approach to the evaluation of organics in drinking water. *U.S.E.P.A.,* 2nd Conference on environmental impact of chlorination, 1977.

12. Rubin, Phillip: Comment: Cancer epidemiology. *JAMA, 226:*1557, 1973.

13. Epidemiology subcommittee of the safe drinking water committee: Epidemiological studies of cancer frequency and certain organic constituents of drinking water. A review of recent published and unpublished literature. *U.S.E.P.A.* by National Academy of Sciences NRC. Wash. D.C. 1978.

14. Ames, Bruce, Durston, Wm. E., Yamasaki, E., and Lee, Frank: Carcinogens are mutagens: a simple test system combining liver homogenates for activation and bacteria for detection. *Proc Nat'l Acad of Sciences, 70:*2281, 1973.

15. McCann, Joyce, Chio, Edw., Yamasaki, Edith, and Ames, Bruce: Detection of carcinogens as mutagens in the *Salmonella*/microsome test: assay of 300 chemicals. *Proc Nat'l Acad of Sciences, 72:*5135, 1975.

16. Fox, Jeffrey L.: Ames test success paves way for short-term cancer testing. *Chem and Eng News,* p. 34, Dec. 12, 1977.

17. Bridges, Bryn A.: Short term screening tests for carcinogens. *Nature, 261:*195, May 20, 1976.

18. Devoret, R.: Bacterial tests for potential carcinogens. *Scientific American, 241 (2):*40, 1979.

19. Smith, Aileen M.: Does the Ames test work? *News Engineer,* p. 25, Apr. 1977.

20. Cairns, Thomas: The ED_{01} study: Introduction, objectives and experimental design. *Env Path and Tox, 3:*1, 1979.

21. National Academy of Sciences-National Research Council, Principles for evaluating environmental chemicals. N.A.S. Wash. D.C. 1977.

22. Jones, T. C.: Mammalian and avian models of disease in man. *Federation Proc, 28(1):*162, 1969.

23. Schein, P., and Anderson, T.: The efficacy of animal studies in predicting clinical toxicity of cancer chemotherapeutic drugs. *J Clin Pharm, 83:*228,

1977.

24. Freireich, Emil., Gehan, Edm. A., Rall, David., Schmidt, Leon., and Skipper, Howard: Quantitative comparison of toxicity of anticancer agents in mouse, rat, dog, monkey, and man. *Cancer Chemotherapy Reports, 50(4):*219, 1966.

25. Baker, S. B. and Davey, O. B.: The predictive value for man of toxicological tests of drugs in laboratory animals. *Br Med Bull, 26(3):*208, 1970.

26. Clegg, D. J.: Animal reproduction and carcinogenicity studies in relation to human safety evaluation. In Deichman, Wm. (Ed.): *Toxicology and Occupational Medicine.* No. Holland, Elsevier, 1979.

27. Jansen, J. D.: The predictive value of tests for carcinogenic and mutagenic activity. In Deichman, Wm. (Ed.): *Toxicology and Occupational Medicine.* No. Holland, Elsevier, 1979.

28. Littlefield, Neil A., Farmer, John, Gaylord, David W., and Sheldon, Winslow G.: Effects of dose and time in a long term-low dose carcinogenic study. *Env Path and Tox, 3:*17, 1979.

29. Pochin, Edw. E.: Assumption of linearity in dose-effect relationships. *Env Health Perspectives, 22:*103, 1978.

30. Saffiotti, U.: Experimental identification of chemical carcinogens, risk evaluation and animal to human correlations. *Env Health Pers, 22:*107, 1978.

31. Guess, H. A., and Crump, K. S.: Best estimate low-dose extrapolation of carcinogenicity data, *Env Health Pers, 22:*149, 1978.

32. Jones, H.: Dose-effect relationships and the matter of threshold of carcinogenesis. *Env Health Pers, 22:*171, 1978.

33. Litchfield, J. T., Jr., and Wilcoxon, F.: A simplified method of evaluating dose effect experiments. *Pharmacology and Experimental Therapeutics, 96:*99, 1949.

34. Schmahl, D.: Problems of dose response studies in chemical carcinogenesis with special reference to n-nitroso compounds. *CRC Crit Rev in Toxicology,* 257, 1979.

35. Mantel, Nathan, Neeit, Bohidar, Brown, Charles C., Ciminera, Joseph L., and Tukey, John: An improved mantel-Bryant procedure for testing of carcinogens. *Cancer Research, 35:*865, 1975.

36. Wilson, Richard: Risks caused by low levels of pollution. *The Yale Journ. of Biol. and Medicine, 51:*37, 1978.

37. Silkworth, J. B., and Loose, L. D.: Environmental chemical induced modification of cell mediated immune responses. *Ann New York Acad Sci,* 1979.

38. Taylor, M. A., Israel, B. A., Escobar, B. R., and Berlinerman, D.: *In vitro* and *in vivo* parameters of humoral and cellular immunity in an animal model for protein calorie malnutrition. *Ann New York Acad Sci,* 1979.

39. Luster, Michael I., Faith, Robt. E., and Clark, George: Laboratory studies on the immune effects of halogenated aromatics. Part VII, Immunologic Abnormalities. *Ann New York Acad Sci,* 1979.

40. Luster, M. I., and Faith.: Assessment of immunologic alterations caused by halogenated hydrocarbons. *Ann New York Acad Sci,* 1979.

41. Dean J. H., Padarathsingh, M. L. and Thomas, J.: Application of immuno-competence assays for defining immunosuppression. *Ann New York Acad Sci,* 1979.

42. Sell, Stewart: Lymphocytes in *Immunology, Immunopathology and Immunity,* 3rd ed. New York, N.Y., Harper and Row, 1980.

43. Drew, I. S.: Immunological surveillance against neoplasia: An immunological quandary. *Human Pathology, 10(1):*5, 1979.

44. Fudenberg, H. H., Stites, D. P., Caldwell, J. S., and Wells, J. V.: *Basic and Clinical Immunology.* Los Altos Calif., Lang Publ. Co., 1980.

45. Benacarraf, B., and Unanue, E.: *Textbook of Immunology.* Baltimore, Williams and Wilkins Publ. Co., 1979.

46. Penn, I.: Cancer associated with immunosuppression. Sect. F. *CRC Handbook* series in clinical laboratory science. Cleveland, Chemical Rubber Publ. Co., 1979.

47. Fraumeni, J. F., and Miller R. W.: Epidemiology of human leukemia. *J Nat Cancer Inst, 38:*593, 1976.

48. McMichael, J. J., Spirtas, P., Kupper, L. L., and Gamble, J. F.: Solvent exposure and leukemia among rubber workers: an epidemiologic study. *Occ. Medicine, 17(4):* 1975.

49. Vigliani, E. C., and Saita G.: Benzene and leukemia. *New Engl J Med, 271:*872, 1964.

50. Infante, P., Rinsky, R. A., Wagoner, J. K., and Young, R. J.: Leukemia in benzene workers. *J Env Path and Toxicology, 2:*251, 1977.

51. Goldstein, B. D.: Hematotoxicity in Humans. *J Tox and Env Health,* Supplement 2, 69, 1977.

52. Forni, A., Pacificao, E., and Limonata, A.: Chromosome studies in workers exposed to benzene, toluene or both. *Arch Env Health, 22:*373, 1971.

53. Maltoni, C. and Scarnato, C.: First experimental demonstration of the carcinogenic effects of benzene. *Med. Lavoro, 70(5):*352, 1979.

54. Wolman, S.: Cytologic and cytogenetic effects of benzene. *J Tox and Env Health,* Supp #2, p. 33, 1977.

55. Picciano, D.: Cytogenetic study of workers exposed to benzene. *Env Res, 19:*33, 1979.

56. Fredman, M. L.: The molecular site of benzene toxicity. *J Tox and Env Health,* Suppl. #2, p. 37, 1977.

57. Zarrabi, M. H., Zucker, S., Miller, F., Cerman, R. M., Romano, G. S., Hartnett, J. A., and Varna, A. O.: Immunologic and coagulation disorders in chlorpromazine treated patients. *Ann of Int Med, 91:*194, 1979.

58. Fidler, I. J.: Depression of macrophages in mice drinking hyperchlorinated water. *Nature, 270(5639):*735, 1977.

59. Hibbs, J. B., and Weinberg J. B.: Suppression of macrophages by chlorinated compounds. *Nature, 269:*245, 1977.

60. Dandliker, W. B., Hicks, A. N., Levison, S. A., Stewart, K., and Brawn, J.: Effects of pesticides on the immune response. *Environmental Sci and Tech, 14(2):*204, 1980.

61. Ceglowski, W. S., Ercegovich, C. D., and Pearson, N. S.: *Lymphocytes and Macrophages,* New York, Plenum Press, 1978.

62. Faith, R. E. and Luster, M.: Investigations on the effects of 2,3,7,8-tetrachlorodibenzodioxin (TCDD) on parameters of various immune functions. *Ann N Y Acad of Sci,* 1979.

63. Thigpen, J. E., Faith, R. F., McConnell, F. F., and Moore, J. A.: Increased susceptibility to bacterial infection as a sequelae of exposure to 2,3,7,8-tetrachlorodibenzodioxin. *Infection and Immunity, 12;* (6) 1319, 1975.

64. Luster, M. I., Clark, G., Lawson, L. D., and Faith, R. E.: Effects of brief *in vitro* exposure to 2,3,7,8-tetrachlorodibenzodioxin on mouse lymphocytes. *J Env Path and Tox,* 2:965, 1979.

65. Sharma, R. P., and Gehring, P.: Effects of 2,3,7,8-tetrachlorodibenzodioxin on splenic lymphocyte transformation in mice after single and repeated exposures. *Ann N Y Acad Sci,* 1979.

66. LaVia, M. F., Loose, L. D., LaVia, D. S., and Silberman, M. S.: The immunosuppressive effect of phenol derivatives. In *Lymphocytes and Macrophages,* New York, Plenum Press, 1978.

67. Oehme, F. W.: Twenty First Gaines Veterinarian Symposium, 1972.

68. Archer, D., Bukovic-Wess, J., and Smith, B.: Immunosuppression by phenol derivatives. *Proc Soc Exp Biol and Med, 156:*465, 1977.

69. Seinen, W., and Penninks, A.: Immune suppression as a consequence of a selective cytotoxic activity of certain organometallic compounds on thymus and thymus dependent lymphocytes. *Ann New York Acad Sci,* 1979.

70. Koller, L. D.: Immunosuppression produced by lead, cadmium and mercury. *Am J Vet Res, 34:*1457, 1973.

71. Koller, L. D., and Kovacic, S.: Decreased antibody formation in mice exposed to lead. *Nature, 250:*148, 1974.

72. Faith, R. E., Luster, M. I., and Kimmel, C. A.: Effect of chronic developmental lead exposure on cell mediated immune functions. *Clin Exp Immunol, 35:*413, 1979.

73. Luster, M. Faith, R. E., and Kimmel, C. A.: Depression of humoral immunity in rats following chronic developmental lead exposure. *Env Path and Tox, 1:*397, 1978.

74. Hoffman, D. J., and Niyogi, S. K.: Metal mutagens and carcinogens affect RNA synthesis rates in a distinct manner. *Science, 198:*513, 1977.

75. Vos, J. G., Van Logten, M. J., Kreeftenberg, J. G., and Kruizinga, W.: Hexachlorobenzene induced stimulation of the humoral immune response in rats. *Ann New York Acad Sci,* 1979.

76. Sharma, R. P., and Gehring, P. J.: Immunologic effects of vinyl chloride in mice. *Ann New York Acad Sci,* 1979.

77. Miller, K.: The effects of asbestos on macrophages. *CRC Critical Reviews in Toxicology,* Sept., 1978.

78. Kagan, E., and Miller, K.: Alveolar macrophage-splenic lymphocyte interactions following chronic asbestos inhalation in the rat. In *Lymphocytes and Macrophages.* New York, Plenum Press, 1978.

79. Herscowitz, H. B., Conrad, R. E., and Pennline, K. H.: Alveolar macrophage-induced suppression of the immune response. In *Lymphocytes and Macrophages.* New York, Plenum Press, 1978.
80. Drath, D. B., Davies, M. L., Karnovsky, M. L., and Huber, G. L.: Tobacco smoke and the pulmonary alveolar macrophage. In *Lymphocytes and Macrophages.* New York, Plenum Press. 1978.
81. Kersey, J. H., Perry, G. S., and Spector, B. D.: Cancer associated with immune deficiency diseases. *CRC Handbook series in Clinical Laboratory Science.* Sect. F. Immunology. Cleveland Ohio, CRC Press, 1978.

Chapter 6

ANIMAL MODEL STUDIES OF PULMONARY RESPONSES

MERYL H. KAROL

Introduction

Inhalation of airborne chemicals may result in a number of adverse pulmonary responses. Depending upon such factors as size of particle, chemical reactivity, and concentration to name a few, respiratory responses may include sensory irritation, pulmonary irritation, and/or pulmonary sensitization. Some generalizations can be made regarding structural features of molecules frequently associated with such adverse responses, but quantitative prediction of irritant or sensitizing abilities of chemicals is based on data collected from animal models. An animal model for sensory irritation, using Swiss-Webster mice was developed several years ago.[1] The correlation between the irritancy of chemicals in the mouse and that reported in the literature for humans has been very high.[2] Thus, this model is well-developed for prediction of irritation abilities of new chemicals for man. In contrast, this laboratory has reported[3] only recently the development of a guinea pig model for pulmonary sensitivity where animals are sensitized by inhalation of small reactive organic chemicals. Procedures have since been developed for screening new chemicals not only for immediate-onset sensitizing abilities, both also for their ability to produce delayed-onset pulmonary hypersensitivity. These developments will be discussed in this report.

Characteristics of Pulmonary Sensitivity

In man, immunologic pulmonary sensitivity is defined as widespread reversible airways obstruction caused by prior exposure to

Written under support from grant #ES01532 from the National Institute of Environmental Health Sciences.

the offending agent. The sensitivity is therefore acquired, occurring only after previous exposure, and is highly specific. Pulmonary reactions may occur during exposure or within an hour of exposure. These reactions are called "immediate" hypersensitivity and have been associated with an IgE or IgG-STS antibody pathogenesis.[4] Alternatively, onset of reactions may begin several hours to one day following exposure. The pathogenesis of this "delayed-onset" response is less clear, but appears to involve, in part, cellular components of the immune system.

An animal model for pulmonary sensitivity must be able to display both types of pulmonary responses. The guinea pig was selected as an animal model for human pulmonary sensitivity because it undergoes pulmonary reactions similar to these seen in humans. The immunologic airways response in the guinea pig is typified by the following characteristics: increased breathing rate, decreased tidal volume, and in severe cases, bronchoconstriction. Typical reaction patterns are shown in Figure 6–1. The degree of respiratory tract sensitivity can be calculated from the observed breathing rate.

Calculation of "Immediate" Respiratory Hypersensitivity

The severity of the respiratory reaction can be determined by calculation of the percent increase in respiratory rate of the guinea pig during inhalation of the allergen compared with the respiratory rate prior to exposure. For this measurement, animals are placed in individual body plethysmographs. Four such plethysmographs are connected to a 10 liter Plexiglass inhalation chamber as shown in Figure 6–2. Air is drawn through the chamber at a rate of 20 l/min. Prior to inhalation of the allergen, the respiratory rate of each animal is measured by use of a pressure transducer connected to the plethysmograph. Signals are converted into electrical output then amplified and displayed on an oscillograph. In this way, each breath of the animal is sensed and recorded. A significant increase in breathing rate during exposure, lasting a minimum of three minutes, is indicative of pulmonary sensitivity.[5]

Protocol for Screening Chemicals

The procedure developed to screen small chemicals for pulmonary sensitizing ability was designed to answer the following questions:

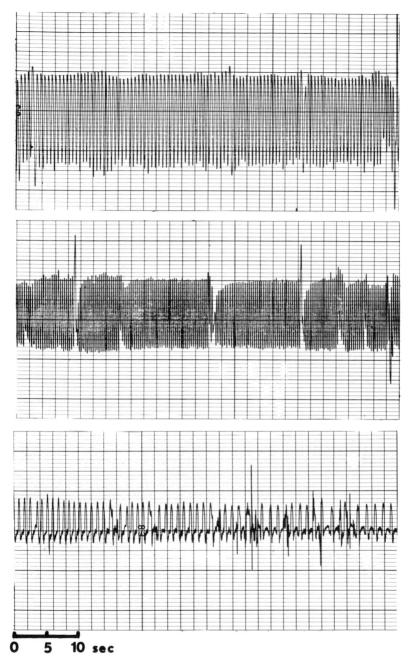

0 5 10 sec

Figure 6–1: Oscillograph display showing respiratory pattern of a single guinea pig before challenge (upper) and during aerosol challenge (middle). Lower pattern indicative of bronchoconstriction.

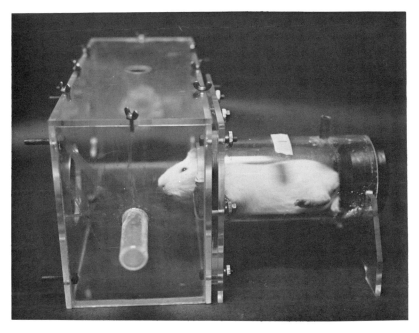

Figure 6–2: Inhalation chamber used for "head only" exposure of guinea pigs and body plethysmographs for measurement of immediate-onset pulmonary sensitivity reactions.

1. Is the chemical recognized as an antigenic determinant?
2. Does pulmonary sensitivity develop as a result of inhalation exposure?
3. Does the agent stimulate a specific antibody response?

Is the Chemical Recognized as an Antigenic Determinant?

Most airborne chemicals of interest in the industrial or environmental setting as pulmonary sensitizers are of low molecular weight. Examples of such compounds include formaldehyde, acrylonitrile and toluene diisocyanate. To test for antigenicity of these substances, while avoiding difficulty which may result from solubility, irritancy or extreme chemical reactivity of some industrial chemicals, hapten-protein conjugates are used for preliminary studies. The chemical of interest assumes the role of hapten, and a protein, frequently ovalbumin, is used as the carrier protein. Guinea pigs are immunized by intraperitoneal injection of the conjugate. Animals are bled fourteen days after and the serum tested for the presence of anti-hapten antibodies.

At least two methods are used to detect antibodies. For a rapid evaluation, double diffusion in gel is employed. Test antigens include (1) the immunizing hapten-protein conjugate, (2) the protein component alone, (3) a second hapten-protein conjugate in which the protein is of guinea pig origin (usually guinea pig serum albumin). A second more specific assay (passive cutaneous anaphylaxis, PCA) is then employed to assess the presence of hapten-specific cytophilic antibodies. These antibodies would more likely be those involved in hypersensitivity reactions.

ANTI–HAPTEN LUNG SENSITIVITY. To determine the presence of anti-hapten sensitivity in the respiratory tract, sensitized animals are tested by bronchial provocation challenge using both the hapten-protein conjugate as well as the chemical hapten itself.

Challenges are performed two to three weeks following immunization. Typically, guinea pigs are challenged by inhalation of hapten-GSA aerosols for ten minutes. Comparison of respiratory rate during exposure with that prior to exposure indicates the presence of hapten-specific pulmonary sensitivity. To assure that sensitivity is not directed toward the protein, animals are challenged with aerosols containing just the protein carrier. These challenges precede those with hapten-conjugates. If carrier-specific sensitivity is present, use of a different protein for conjugate formation is indicated.

Hapten-specific lung sensitivity is also assessed by inhalation challenge with hapten alone. Frequently, in these instances, care must be taken to generate a concentration of the chemical that is not irritating. It would be expected that animals possessing hapten-specific pulmonary sensitivity would respond to challenge with both hapten-conjugate and hapten alone. However, from studies with TDI sensitivity, animals usually showed greater response when challenged with the hapten-conjugate as compared with hapten alone.

Does Pulmonary Sensitization Result from Inhalation Exposure?

To determine if inhalation exposure can result in hapten specific pulmonary hypersensitivity, guinea pigs are sensitized using a "head only" exposure. Pigs are restrained in body plethysmographs during exposures. To sensitize with hapten-protein conjugates, animals are routinely exposed to aerosols of conjugate for 10 minutes a day on five consecutive days. Fourteen days later, sensitivity is assessed by aerosol challenge and serologic assay. This procedure has been used to produce pulmonary sensitivity to the following haptens: p-tolyl isocyanate,[5] p-azobenzene arsonate,[5] and hexyl isocyanate.[6]

Pulmonary sensitivity as a result of inhalation of a chemical has been achieved to date with just two chemicals: p-tolyl isocyanate[3] and toluene diisocyanate.[3] With both chemicals, pulmonary sensitivity, as well as the antibody response, was dose-dependent. High concentrations succeeded in sensitizing a greater number of animals and resulted in generally higher antibody titers than did exposure to low concentrations of chemicals.

DELAYED–ONSET PULMONARY SENSITIVITY. Not infrequently, pulmonary sensitivity responses occur several hours following exposure. Such responses may be difficult to relate to the particular exposure. The following substances have been associated with delayed reactions: formaldehyde, TDI, trimellitic anhydride, as well as other environmental agents. Symptoms in man include chest tightness, difficulty breathing, malaise, and occasionally fever. Reactions may start one hour after exposure or several hours from exposure and last for hours.

Total evaluation of the pulmonary sensitizing ability of chemicals must include consideration of delayed reactions. Because animals cannot be restrained for long periods, the body plethysmograph used to measure immediate reactions cannot be used for delayed-onset reactions. For this reason an alternative plethysmograph was developed[7] that allows guinea pigs complete freedom to move, eat, or sleep while permitting measurement of respiratory rate and breathing pattern. The design is based on a previous chamber developed by Jacky.[8] The chamber was found capable of detecting a delayed-onset pulmonary reaction in the following experiment. Guinea pigs were sensitized by injection of Freund's adjuvant and challenged three weeks later by inhalation of purified protein derivative (PPD). No respiratory responses were observed during exposure. However, six to eight hours following inhalation challenge, a gradual increase in respiratory rates was noted that lasted several hours. Increases were 50 to 70 percent above prechallenge breathing rates. The immunologic nature of the responses was apparent from histologic examination of lung tissue. Predominant in these sections was infiltration of mononuclear cells into alveolar spaces and perivascular involvement. These reactions were not observed in lung tissue from control animals exposed to PPD aerosol.

The development of a method to continually monitor the respiratory rates in guinea pigs for periods up to forty-eight hours should permit evaluation of the total hypersensitivity lung response to inhaled both agents including immediate and delayed onset reactions.

Does the Agent Stimulate A Specific Antibody Response?

Both immediate and delayed-onset pulmonary hypersensitivity responses have been associated with immunologic mechanisms. As part of the procedure to evaluate materials for pulmonary sensitizing ability, the presence of an antibody response is explored. Animals are bled two weeks following exposure and serum evaluated for hapten-specific antibodies as described above. The presence of cytophilic antibodies in the serum indicates exposure to the specific agent, but does not necessarily imply the presence of pulmonary sensitivity to the agent.[3]

Relationship of Dermal and Pulmonary Sensitivity

In order to avoid the complexities of testing for pulmonary sensitivity as detailed above, the possibility of employing a skin test to indicate the existence of pulmonary sensitivity was explored.[9] Guinea pigs were sensitized to dinitrochlorobenzene (DNCB) by topical application. Seven days later, skin tests revealed the presence of delayed dermal sensitivity to DNCB. Bronchial provocation challenge with DNCB however failed to evoke a delayed pulmonary response. Similarly bronchial provocation challenge with a DNCB-protein conjugate also yielded negative results. Thus, the relationship, if any, between specific delayed dermal reactivity and respiratory tract reactivity remains to be elucidated.

Conclusions

The ability of various environmental and industrial agents to cause hypersensitivity of the respiratory tract is unquestioned. Animal models of pulmonary sensitivity can be of great value in predicting and evaluating pulmonary sensitizing abilities of varied materials. In guinea pigs, dermal sensitivity and antibody titers to specific chemicals cannot be used to predict lung sensitivity. However, measurement of immediate and delayed pulmonary sensitivity reactions in guinea pig models offers great promise for evaluation of the sensitizing potencies of various chemicals toward the respiratory tract.

References

1. Alarie, Y.: Irritating properties of airborne materials to the upper respiratory tract. *Arch Environ Health, 13:*433–449, 1966.
2. Alarie, Y.: Dose-response analysis in animal studies: Prediction of human responses. *Environ Health Perspect* (in press).
3. Karol, M. H., Dixon, C., Brady, M., and Alarie, Y.: Immunologic sensitization and pulmonary hypersensitivity by repeated inhalation of aromatic isocyanates. *Toxicol Appl Pharmacol, 53:*260–270, 1980.
4. Pepys, J.: Occupational asthma: Review of present clinical and immunologic status. *J Allergy Clin Immunol, 66:*179–185, 1980.
5. Karol, M. H., Ioset, H., Riley, E. J., and Alarie, Y.: Hapten-specific respiratory hypersensitivity in guinea pigs. *Am Ind Hyg Assoc J, 39:*546–556, 1978.
6. Karol, M. H., Hauth, B., and Alarie, Y.: Pulmonary hypersensitivity to hexyl isocyanate-ovalbumin aerosol in guinea pigs. *Toxicol Appl Pharmacol, 51:*73–80, 1979.
7. Karol, M. H., Underhill, D., Stadler, J., and Alarie, Y.: Monitoring delayed respiratory hypersensitivity in guinea pigs. *Society of Toxicology,* Annual Meeting, 1981.
8. Jacky, J.: A plethysmograph for long-term measurements of ventilation in unrestrained animals. *J Appl Physiol: Respirat Environ Exercise Physiol, 45(4):*664–647, 1978.
9. Stadler, J. and Karol, M., unpublished data.

Chapter 7

CHEMICAL MUTAGENS AND CARCINOGENS IN THE ENVIRONMENT

MICHAEL J. PLEWA

Introduction

The Problem

This lecture is but the briefest of introductions into a novel area of toxicology, that of genetic toxicology. The departure of this field from classical toxicology is manifested by the fact that the focus of the effects of genetic toxins upon the public health does not have a generational endpoint. In other words, agents that cause damage to genes, the units of heredity, can exert detrimental biological effects upon an individual and also upon his offspring. Therefore, the death of an affected individual is no longer the ultimate and worst case of a toxin. It is an inherent and primary responsibility of the present generation to insure the vitality and stability of the human population by the successful transmission of an undamaged genome to the future members of our species. The genetic heritage of mankind defined in our genome is now at risk! The chronic exposure of large populations to genetic toxins in our environment (environmental mutagens) and their consequent effects has become a significant public health problem.

An environmental mutagen is a physical or chemical agent released into the environment that can alter the genome or the proper functioning of the genome. The presence of such genotoxic agents in the environment is a serious threat to the public health.[1-8] Depending upon the ontogenetic stage of an organism, an environmental mutagen may exert teratogenic effects, affect the aging process, induce mutations that involve germinal cells,[9-11] precipitate coronary disease[12] or cause mutations that lead to cancer.[8,13-17] Genetic assays have been developed to determine the mutagenic properties of chemicals. The approach to reduce the impact of environmental mutagens upon the public health is simply to reduce the exposure of people to such agents. The role of regulating the release of toxic chemicals into the environment is a responsibility of the United States Environmental Protection Agency. The enforcement powers of such regulation are derived from federal statutes such as the Toxic Substances Control Act, the Resource Conservation and Recovery Act and the Clean Air and Clean Water Acts. Environmental mutagens are defined as toxins (genotoxins) and, thus, are under the control of several federal and state agencies. However, a battery of good and quantitative genetic assays must be used to adequately determine the genotoxic properties of chemicals, combinations of chemicals and complex environmental pollutants.

We have become aware during the last decade that a number of widely used chemicals possess mutagenic and carcinogenic properties. However, the production, use and human exposure to a great variety of largely untested synthetic organic compounds is a relatively recent event in our history. The annual production of synthetic compounds in the United States has risen from approximately 4.5×10^8 kg in 1940 to approximately 1.4×10^{11} kg in 1976.[18] These chemicals include industrial products and solvents, fuels, agricultural chemicals, drugs, and consumer products. All of us have benefited by this production in terms of our increased standard of living. Items that we consider ordinary, even necessities, were undreamed of in 1930. However, we as individuals and as a society must pay a price for our high living standards, and only now is the toxicological price tag becoming apparent. One currency that is being paid is manifested in our rising cancer rates.[19,20]

This rapid rise in the amounts of chemicals that modern society produces and consumes has inadvertently increased our risk to cancer simply because some widely used agents cause cancer. A partial list of agents that induce cancer in humans and/or in laboratory animals is presented in Table 7–I. The disturbing fact is that the production and use of these agents are generally increasing year after year. In a lecture presented at the University of Illinois, Doctor Bruce Ames stressed the increased production of 1,2 dichloroethane and vinyl chloride during the last decade.[8] Both chemicals are mutagenic and carcinogenic. It is not just industrial chemicals that pose a genotoxic hazard. Increasing amounts of agricultural pesticides, some of which are mutagens and carcinogens, are being used each year. In Table 7–II, a list of pesticides that have been tested by the National Cancer Institute is presented. Occupational exposure to these chemicals as well as exposure to pesticide residues in the food chain may pose a public health hazard.

The Spectrum of Genetic Damage

Chemical environmental mutagens are serious threats because of their ability to induce damage in the genetic material, deoxyribonucleic acid (DNA). DNA is the chemical thread that unites all 132 life forms from bacteria to man. Agents that can damage DNA in one type of organism have a high probability of causing DNA damage in other organisms. Chemical mutagens that induce damage in bacteria, fruit flies, maize, and mice will probably do so in man.

There is a spectrum of genetic damage that is generically referred to as mutation. I shall briefly describe various types of mutation,

Table 7–I

PARTIAL LIST OF CHEMICAL CARCINOGENS

Asbestos
2-Acetylaminofluorene
4-Aminobiphenyl
Benzene
Benzidine
Cadmium
Bischloromethylether
Chloramphenicol
Cyclophosphamide
Diethylstilbestrol
Vinyl chloride
Beta-propiolactone
Beta-naphthylamine
Ethyleneimine
Chloromethylmethylether
4-Nitrobiphenyl
N-Nitrosodimethylamine
coal tars
cigarette smoke

Adapted from S. S. Epstein: *The Politics of Cancer.* New York, Anchor Press/Doubleday, 1979.

Table 7–II

NATIONAL CANCER INSTITUTE
TESTS FOR CARCINOGENICITY OF PESTICIDES

Common or Trade Name	Result
HERBICIDES	
Chloramiben	+
Nitrofen	+
Sulfallate	+
Trifluralin	+
INSECTICIDES	
Dichlorvos	±
Endosulfan	−
Endrin	−
Malathion	−
Methoxychlor	−
Parathion	−
Aldrin	+
Chlordane	+
Kepone	+
Dieldrin	+
Heptachlor	+
Tetrachlorvinphos	+
Toxaphene	+
FUNGICIDES	
Captan	+
PCNB	−
ACARICIDES	
Chlorobenzilate	+
Dicofol	+
Dimethoate	−
Lindane	−
FUMIGANTS	
Dibromochloropropane	+
1, 2-dibromoethane	+
Chloropicrin	−

+ Positive carcinogenic properties when tested on rodents.
− Negative carcinogenic properties when tested on rodents.
± Weakly positive carcinogenic response or conflicting data.

because I want to emphasize that there is a wide variety of different types of genetic damage and exposure to a mutagen can cause more than one type of insult to the genome. Genetic damage may be broadly divided into two major categories: chromosomal effects and point mutations. Changes in the chromosome number or ploidy usually induces genic imbalances. Chromosomal aberrations consist primarily of chromosome breaks, deletions, duplications, inversions and translocations. These chromosomal alterations can be viewed by microscopic examination of affected cells. Point mutations may be easily defined as single gene mutations and consist of base pair substitutions and of additions or deletions of base pairs in DNA. Both types of genetic damage, that to chromosomes and to single genes, pose a danger not only to humans but to all life forms.

Mutation is one source of genetic variation, and it is variation that provides the steam to move the engine of evolution. However, the rate of change of a gene is a characteristic that has evolved. We now are in an era where this rate can be accelerated because of environmental pollutants. I can reasonably speculate that our increased exposure to chemical mutagens will result in an increase in the rates of genetic disease and cancer.

Relationship Between Mutagenesis and Carcinogenesis

A series of recent studies has clearly demonstrated that a high correlation exists between carcinogenic and mutagenic activity of chemicals. In a study involving 300 chemicals, Doctor Ames and his colleagues reported 90 percent of the known carcinogens were mutagenic in the bacterium *Salmonella typhimurium*.[21,22] In a study involving over 600 chemicals conducted in Japan by Doctor Sugimura's laboratory, 85 percent of the carcinogens were also mutagenic.[23] In another independent investigation conducted in Great Britain by Imperial Chemical Industries, 120 chemicals were evaluated and 93 percent of the carcinogens also induced mutation.[24] Many scientists now believe that carcinogens cause cancer because of their mutagenic properties. The somatic mutation theory of cancer suggests that cancer is caused by environmental mutagens.[8] There is a wealth of supporting evidence for the validity of this theory. Epidemiological studies indicate that there exists a twenty to thirty year latent period between exposure to a carcinogen and the appearance of most forms of human cancer.[25] It is tempting and yet reasonable to hypothesize that the rise in the cancer rates that we are currently experiencing is due to the exposure of people to mutagens in the 1950s. However, I must emphasize that environmental mutagens do not pose a hazard just because they are carcinogenic, but because they are mutagenic. A prudent course of action to reduce the hazards to the public health posed by mutagens is to prevent the public from being exposed to these agents.

USEPA Phased Testing Strategy

The United States Environmental Protection Agency has published a phased testing strategy for the analysis of genotoxic chemicals.[26] The strategy consists of three phases: (1) the detection of a genotoxic hazard, (2) confirmation of mutagenic activity in other test systems and the delineation of hazard type, and (3) final determination of the spectrum of genetic effects produced and an assessment of the risks to man. The first phase usually encompasses the use of short-term bacterial assays for mutagenic activity. The most popular genetic assay was developed by Doctor Ames and is based on various histidine-requiring strains of *Salmonella*. In addition, short-term assays to measure primary DNA damage in bacteria and tests that measure chromosome effects in cultured cells are included in the first phase. In phase one, *in vitro* activation methods are used to determine if metabolism of the test agent can convert it into a mutagen. The most widely used *in vitro* activation system uses microsomes prepared from rat liver. However, other activation systems including plant systems are now being developed.[27,28] In phase two, chemicals that elicit a positive response in phase one tests are evaluated with short-term assays that involve mammalian cells, insects, and plants. These tests verify the mutagenic properties of the agent and help define the range of genetic damage induced. The final phase of testing, phase three, includes the testing of the chemical in whole animals. These tests are expensive, costing $300,000 or more and require several years to complete. These phase three studies establish the final validation of hazard and provide an assessment of risk.

Scientists are now trying to assess the risks to humans posed by exposure to environmental mutagens. A recent publication, The Banbury Report, 1 *Assessing Chemical Mutagens: The Risk to Humans*, is devoted entirely to the subject of risk assessment.[29] A good approach to calibrate the risk of exposure to a chemical mutagen is to relate the amount of mutation caused by a chemical to an equivalent amount of damage induced by ionizing radiation. Such a unit of risk measurement is defined as a radiation equivalent chemical or REC.[6] It is hoped that adequate strategies for risk assessment can be developed so that the empirical data derived from the laboratory can be used in calculating the risk vs. benefit relationship for each chemical.

Conclusion

In conclusion, we are constantly being exposed to a wide variety of genetically active agents. It is the role of the genetic toxicologist to detect these agents and ascertain their degree of risk. In an effort to protect the public health, regulatory agencies must then use this information to set limits of exposure under occupational settings and for the general population.

REFERENCES

1. Abrahamson, S.: Comments on and summary of panel on assessment of *in vitro* and *in vivo* mutagenicity data with regard to safety evaluation. *Environ Health Perspect, 6:*193–194, 1973.
2. Legator, M. S., and Flamm, W. G.: Environmental mutagenesis and repair. *Ann Rev Biochem, 42:*683–708, 1973.
3. de Serres, F. J.: The utility of short-term tests for mutagenicity in the toxicological evaluation of environmental agents. *Mutat Res, 33:*11–15, 1975.
4. de Serres, F. J.: Mutagenicity of chemical carcinogens. *Mutat Res, 41:*43–50, 1976.
5. de Serres, F. J.: Problems associated with the application of short-term tests for mutagenicity in mass-screening programs. *Environ Mutagenesis, 1:*203–208, 1979.
6. Drake, J. W., Abrahamson, S., Crow, J. F., Hollaender, A., Lederberg, S., Legator, M. S., Neel, J. V., Shaw, M. W., Sutton, H. E., Von Borstel, R. C., and Zimmering, S.: Environmental mutagenic hazards. *Science, 187:*503–514, 1975.
7. Bartsch, H.: Predictive value of mutagenicity tests in chemical carcinogenesis. *Mutat Res, 38:*177–190, 1976.
8. Ames, B. N.: Identifying environmental chemicals causing mutations and cancer. *Science, 204:*587–593, 1979.

9. Crow, J. F.: Impact of various types of genetic damage and risk assessment. *Environ Health Perspect*, 6:1–5, 1973.

10. Freese, E.: Thresholds in toxic, teratogenic, mutagenic, and carcinogenic effects. *Environ Health Perspect*, 6:171–178, 1973.

11. Freese, E.: Genetic effects of mutagens and of agents present in the human environment. In Prakash, L. (Ed.): *Molecular and Environmental Aspects of Mutagenesis*. Springfield, Thomas, 1974, pp. 5–13.

12. Benditt, E. P.: The origin of atherosclerosis. *Scientific Am*, 236:74–85, 1977.

13. Bouck, N., and di Mayorca, G.: Somatic mutation as the basis for malignant transformation of BHK cells by chemical carcinogens. *Nature*, 264:722–727, 1976.

14. Cairns, J.: The cancer problem. *Scientific Am*, 233:64–78, 1975.

15. Cairns, J.: Mutation selection and the natural history of cancer. *Nature*, 255:197–200, 1975.

16. de Serres, F. J.: The correlation between carcinogenic and mutagenic activity in short-term tests for mutation-induction and DNA repair. *Mutat Res*, 31:203–204, 1975.

17. Miller, E. C., and Miller, J. A.: The mutagenicity of chemical carcinogens: correlations, problems and interpretations. In Holleander, A. (Ed.): *Chemical Mutagens: Principles and Methods for Their Detection*. New York, Plenum Press, 1971, pp. 83–119.

18. U.S. International Trade Commission, (1978).

19. Pollack, E. S., and Horm, J. W.: Trends in cancer incidence and the United States, 1969–76. *J Natl Cancer Inst*, 64:1091–1103, 1980.

20. Epstein, S. S.: *The Politics of Cancer*. New York, Anchor Press/Doubleday, 1979, 628 pp.

21. McCann, J., Choi, E., Yamasaki, E., and Ames, B. N.: Detection of carcinogens as mutagens in the *Salmonella*/microsome test: assay of 300 chemicals. *Proc Natl Acad Sci USA*, 72:5135–5139, 1975.

22. McCann, J., and Ames, B. N.: Detection of carcinogens as mutagens in the *Salmonella*/microsome test: assay of 300 chemicals. Part II. *Proc Natl Acad Sci USA*, 73:950–954, 1976.

23. Sugimura, T., Sato, S., Nagao, M., Yahaggi, T., Matsushima, T., Seino, Y., Takeuchi, M., and Kawachi, T.: Overlapping of carcinogens and mutagens. In Magee, P. B. (Ed.): *Fundamentals in Cancer Prevention*. Baltimore, MD, University Park Press, 1976, pp. 191–215.

24. Purchase, I. F. H., Longstaff, E., Ashby, J., Styles, J. A., Anderson, D., Lefevre, P. A., and Westwood, F. R.: Evaluation of six short-term tests for potential carcinogenicity and recommendations for their use. *Nature*, 264:624–627, 1976.

25. Cairns, J.: *Cancer, Science and Society*. San Francisco, CA, W. H. Freeman and Co., 1978.

26. Trontell, A.: Environmental assessment: Short-term tests for carcinogens, mutagens and other genotoxic agents. *Technology Transfer*, EPA–625/9–79–003, 1979.

27. Plewa, M. J.: Activation of chemicals into mutagens by green plants: A preliminary discussion. *Environ Health Perspect, 27:*45–50, 1978.

28. Plewa, M. J., and Gentile, J. M.: The activation of chemicals into mutagens by green plants. In de Serres, F. J. (Ed.): *Chemical Mutagens: Principles and Methods for their Detection.* New York, Plenum Press, IN PRESS.

29. McElheny, V. K., and Abrahamson, S.: *Banbury Report 1. Assessing Chemical Mutagens: The Risks to Humans.* Cold Spring Harbor, NY, Cold Spring Harbor Laboratory, 1979.

Chapter 8

HOW TO MAKE AN "EDUCATED GUESS" ABOUT THE TERATOGENICITY OF CHEMICAL COMPOUNDS

Vera Kolb Meyers and Roger E. Beyler

Teratogens* are agents that act during pregnancy to produce a physical or functional defect in the embryo, fetus, or offspring (1). Teratogens may be chemicals, viruses, or physical factors (e.g. X-ray radiation, etc.) (1). The vast majority of teratogens are chemicals: drugs, agricultural chemicals, common solvents, and reagents (2). Since practising chemists spend a good share of their lives in the laboratory in contact with chemicals, they need to be able to do the following: (a) recognize known teratogens; (b) predict teratogenicity of a compound that has not been tested; and (c) protect themselves from proven or suspected teratogens. The objective of this chapter is to briefly discuss these three points, with an emphasis on the ability to predict teratogenicity.

Information on Known Teratogens

Known teratogens are described in the *Registry of Toxic Effects of Chemical Substances* (RTECS) (3) or in its subfile of "Tumorigenic, Teratogenic and Mutagenic Citations" (4). A list of 527 teratogenic substances obtained by computer search of RTECS has been published (2). Evidence for teratogenicity of substances listed in RTECS is based primarily on animal data and is unevaluated (3).

It should be emphasized that prediction of teratogenicity of chemicals in humans which is based only on animal studies is often very poor (5).

---

*The word *teratogen* is derived from the Greek word *teratos* meaning monster and *gene* meaning forming.

Prediction of Teratogenicity of New Compounds

Ideally, a chemist should be able to make a scientifically sound prediction about the teratogenicity of a chemical just by looking at its structure. Such predictions would be based on a thorough understanding of the mechanism of action (6) and structure-activity relationships of teratogens (7). In reality, however, this is not possible because at this time we have only a very limited knowledge of these (6,7). What chemists can do at the present time, however, is first to become informed about the chemical structures and the biological activities displayed most often by the known teratogens; then, on the basis of these data, chemists should make an "educated guess" about the teratogenicity of a new compound.

Chemical structures of most teratogenic substances in the list of 527 cited above (2) are known and were identified by a time-consuming process, since both IUPAC nomenclature and common names were used. Structural formulas of teratogens were drawn* following IUPAC nomenclature rules (8–10) in the former case, and the Merck Index (11) in the latter case. Careful investigation of these structures revealed that most teratogens display the chemical structures presented in Table 8–I.

Table 8–I

CLASSIFICATION OF TERATOGENS BY CHEMICAL STRUCTURES

Acrylates
Alkaloids
Amides
Amines and Ammonium Salts
Azo Compounds
Barbituric Acid Derivatives
Benzodiazepines
Carbamates
Chlorinated Hydrocarbons
Folic Acid Derivatives
Glutamic Acid Derivatives
Hydrazines
Hydantoins
Imides
Indandiones
Metals (Pb, Hg, Cd, As, etc.)
Nitroso Compounds

*These structural formulas are available from the authors at a nominal cost.

Table 8–I Continued

CLASSIFICATION OF TERATOGENS BY CHEMICAL STRUCTURES ›

Phenethylamines
Phenothiazines
Phthalimides
Piperazines
Polynuclear Hydrocarbons
Purines
Pyrimidines
Salicylates
Steroids
Sulfonamides
Tetracyclines
Thiadiazoles
Thiocarbamates
Thiophosphates
Triazenes
Triazines
Ureas

More than half of the 527 teratogens studied show biological activity, most often as drugs for human or animal use or as agricultural chemicals. This was found by consulting of the Merck Index (11). A comprehensive review of the teratogenicity hazard to humans from drugs is provided by the book of Nishimura and Tanimura (12). Classification of teratogens by biological activity is presented in Table 8–II.

The contents of Tables 8–I and 8–II demonstrate that teratogens display a great variety of chemical structures and biological activities in which no simple pattern is obvious. The 527 structures of teratogens do not appear to be a suitable data set for pattern recognition analysis (13). The reason is simply that not *all* of these structures are necessarily *recognized* by the receptors, enzymes, or sense organs of the embryo or fetus in a fashion in which, for example, estrogens are recognized by the estrogen receptors (14) or opiates by the opiate receptors (15). The "structurally specific"† teratogens, whose activity results essentially from their chemical

---

†The division of teratogens into structurally specific and structurally nonspecific classes was done by analogy with drugs (16).

Table 8–II

CLASSIFICATION OF TERATOGENS BY BIOLOGICAL ACTIVITY

Anticoagulants (e.g. coumarins)

Anticonvulsants (barbiturates, hydantoins, oxazolidines, and succinimides)

Antineoplastics (e.g. nitrogen mustards and others alkylating agents, antimetabolites such as purine, pyrimidine, and folic acid antagonists, antibiotics such as actinomycin D, mitomycin C, alkaloids such as colchicine and vincristine)

Cardiovascular Agents (such as vasoconstrictors and vasodilators)

Carcinogenics (azo dyes, nitrosamines, polynuclear hydrocarbons, chlorinated hydrocarbons)

Chelating agents (d-penicillamine, EDTA, BAL)

Chemotherapeutic Agents (such as antibiotics, sulfonamides, quinine and related substances)

CNS Affecting Agents (some anaesthetics, hypnotics, narcotics, sedatives, tranquilizers, analgesics)

Diuretics (xanthines, thiadiazoles)

Hormones and Antihormones (corticosteroids, androgens, progestogens, estrogens, antithyroid drugs, ACTH, epinephrine, insulin and oral hypoglycemics such as sulfonylureas)

Neuropharmacological Agents (such as organophosphorous anticholinesterases like parathion; amphetamines, atropines, ganglion-blocking agents such as tetraethylammonium chloride)

Pesticides (herbicides like 2,4-D and 2,4,5-T; insecticides like carbamates, chlorinated hydrocarbons, thiophosphates; fungicides)

Psychotomimetics (LSD and mescaline)

Vitamins (A and D in high dossage)

---

structure (specific configuration, conformation, and charge distribution) would be recognized. However, the "structurally nonspecific"† teratogens may not be recognized, since their activity does not strictly depend on chemical structure, except to the extent that structure affects physicochemical properties responsible for teratogenicity (e.g. complexing ability, oxidation-reduction potentials, etc.). Since quite different chemical structures may have similar physicochemical properties, and thus a similar teratogenic

---

†The division of teratogens into structurally specific and structurally nonspecific classes was done by analogy with drugs (16).

effect, application of the pattern recognition method for analysis of these structures would not be justified. Unfortunately, the distinction between these two classes of teratogens is not always clear. It appears then that the use of a pattern recognition method for prediction of teratogenicity would not give good correlations within our data set.

One can circumvent, at least partially, the need for distinguishing specific and nonspecific teratogens by considering their biological effects (other than teratogenic) to be the cause for an abnormality in the developing embryo or fetus, as shown in Scheme I. Thus, an antineoplastic action, a change in blood pressure, or an anticonvulsant action, etc., caused by either a specific or nonspecific teratogen (or both), may be considered to be the teratogenic cause (see solid arrows in Scheme I). This assumption, however, is not necessarily valid for all the compounds in our data set. In some instances the teratogenic response may be directly mediated (see dashed arrows in Scheme I for such a direct teratogenic effect).

SCHEME I

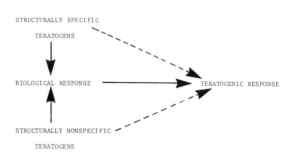

Structure 8–1

Based on our data set and Scheme I, the following procedure is proposed to make an educated guess about teratogenicity of a compound that has not been tested.

1. If the compound in question is a derivative*or a near homo-

---

*The word *derivative* is used by us on the basis of nomenclature found in RTECS, regardless of any other considerations. This means that the alphabetization of names is more important than chemical or biological relationships. Examples (see Appendix I): compound *24* is a derivative of *acetic acid,* compound *106* is a derivative of *butyric acid,* and compound *392* is a derivative of *propionic acid.* None of these are treated as *derivatives* of 2,4,5-trichlorophenol.

log or isostere of a known teratogen (consult Appendixes I and II of this chapter) or if it has a structure displayed by known teratogens (Table 8–I), assume that it is teratogenic. For example, if a compound is an imide, an educated guess would say that it is teratogenic, since many imides (including thalimide) are teratogens. This guess is likely to produce *false positives*, probably more in structurally specific than in structurally nonspecific teratogens.

2. If the compound has the type of biological activity displayed by known teratogens (Table 8–II), assume that it is teratogenic. For example, if the compound is carcinogenic, an educated guess would say that it is also teratogenic, based on the fact that 30 percent of teratogens studied are carcinogens (Appendix I). These guesses are also likely to produce *false positives*, particularly when only a few compounds of a given bioactivity are in the data set.

If both 1 and 2 are applicable to the same compound, it is reasonable to expect that the number of false positives one predicts will be smaller than if only 1 or only 2 are applicable.

An example of the application of this guessing procedure should be of interest. When applied to eighty-six new teratogens (see Appendix II) it was found that seventy of these are derivatives of teratogens in Appendix I, and seven (which are *not* derivatives) have biological activities "characteristic" for teratogens (Table 8–II). Teratogenicity of eight compounds was not obvious: acetaldehyde; 1-adamantanamine hydrochloride; carbon disulfide; ethylene oxide; malonic acid, diethylester; nickel carbonyl; papain; and stannane, hydroxytriphenyl. However, the fact that teratogenicity of seventy-seven compounds out of eighty-six considered (90%) was easily guessed by the above procedure is not necessarily a reflection of reliability in our guessing procedure. Other factors, such as the choice of chemicals for teratogenicity testing may be involved.

Safety Measures for Handling Teratogens

When handling teratogens, chemists should follow safety measures prescribed for working with carcinogens or mutagens (17). Safety precautions should also be taken while working with a compound "guessed" to be teratogenic (*vide supra*). The fact that the above guessing procedure has a built-in characteristic of producing false positives should not represent a serious drawback from the point of view of practising chemists. The reason is simply that chemists as a population group have a very high risk-benefit ratio for exposure to teratogens, as well as other toxic substances. The benefit is greatly enhanced and risk reduced by working under *minimum possible* occupational exposure. Safety precautions taken while working with a compound "guessed" to be teratogenic will definitely reduce the risk if the compound is indeed teratogenic. If the compound is not teratogenic there is little benefit lost in following unnecessary safety measures except perhaps some time and convenience in performing the experiments. Methods used for lowering the risk-benefit ratio, such as using a hood, protective gloves, etc., are not costly at the research lab stage. Of course, they can become more costly at pilot plant and production levels. Even so, the cost in terms of abnormal child care and maintenance, lawsuits by employees, government involvement, etc., demands that exposure to assumed teratogens be minimized.

APPENDIX I

List of Teratogenic Substances*

This list was computer-generated on January 12, 1979, by Medlars II through a search in RTECS. Thanks are expressed to Richard J. Lewis, Sr., and Robert Delmage, both of NIOSH, and to Jean E. Crampon, of the Southern Illinois University Medical Library, who were instrumental in providing us with this information.

The teratogenic substances in this list which are *Category I Carcinogens* or *Suspected Carcinogens* are so denoted. Category I Carcinogens are confirmed carcinogens based on human data or on tests on two mammalian species or on one species if the tests have been replicated. This information was taken from the list of carcinogens published in C&EN, July 31, 1978. The information on suspected carcinogens was taken from the listings in a NIOSH subfile of RTECS entitled "Suspected Carcinogens", 1976.

> Evidence of teratogenicity of substances listed is based on human or animal data.

> The data cited in RTECS, from which this teratogen classification was made, are unevaluated.

TERATOGENIC SUBSTANCES   *NOTE*

(1) Acetamide, N, N-diethyl-
(2) Acetamide, N, N-dimethyl-
(3) Acetamide, N-fluoren-2-yl   Category I carcinogen
(4) Acetamide, N-methyl
(5) Acetamide, N-(2-quinolyl) thio-,
     hydrochloride
(6) Acetamide, N-(5-sulfamoyl-1, 3, 4-
     thiadiazol-2-yl)-
(7) Acetamide, N-(5-sulfamoyl-1, 3, 4-
     thiadiazol-2-yl)-, monosodium salt

*From Vera Kolb Meyers and C. Y. Meyers: *Chemicals Which Cause Birth Defects — Teratogens. A Brief Guide*. Carbondale, IL, Southern Illinois University, 1980. Courtesy of the authors. Reprinted by permission.

TERATOGENIC SUBSTANCES   *NOTE*

(8) Acetanilide, 4'-(bis(2-chloroethyl)
     amino)-
(9) Acetanilide, 4'-(bis(2-chloroethyl)
     amino)-2-fluoro-
(10) Acetic acid, ((4-chloro-o-tolyl)oxy)-,
     ethyl ester
(11) Acetic acid, (2, 4-dichlorophenoxy)-
(12) Acetic acid, (2, 4-dichlorophenoxy)-,
     butoxyethyl ester
(13) Acetic acid, (2, 4-dichlorophenoxy)-,
     butoxypropyl ester
(14) Acetic acid, 2, 4-dichlorophenoxy)-,
     butyl ester
(15) Acetic acid, (2, 4-dichlorophenoxy)-,
     butyl ester and 2, 4, 5-trichloro-
     phenoxyacetic acid (45.5% : 48.2%)
(16) Acetic acid, (2, 4-dichlorophenoxy)-,
     compd. with dimethylamine (1:1)
(17) Acetic acid, (2, 4-dichlorophenoxy)-,
     isooctyl ester   Suspected carcinogen
(18) Acetic acid, (2, 4-dichlorophenoxy)-
     mixed with 2, 4, 5-trichloropheno-
     xyacetic acid (2:1)
(19) Acetic acid, (ethylenedinitrilo)
     tetra-
(20) Acetic acid, (ethylenedinitrilo)
     tetra-, di-sodium salt
(21) Acetic acid, iodo-   Suspected carcinogen
(22) Acetic acid, lead(2+) salt   Category I carcinogen
(23) Acetic acid, mercury(2+) salt
(24) Acetic acid, (2, 4, 5-trichloro-
     phenoxy)-   Suspected carcinogen
(25) Acetic acid, (2, 4, 5-trichloro-
     phenoxy)-, 2-butoxypropyl ester
(26) Acetic acid, (2, 4, 5-trichloro-
     phenoxy)-, butyl ester

TERATOGENIC SUBSTANCES   *NOTE*

(27) Acetic acid, (2, 4, 5-trichloro-
     phenoxy)-, isooctyl ester
(28) Acetohydroxamic acid
(29) Acetonitrile, amino-, bisulfate
(30) Acrylic acid
(31) Acrylonitrile   Suspected carcinogen
(32) Actinomycin D   Suspected carcinogen
(33) Adenine
(34) Adenine, 9-beta-D-arabinofuranosyl-
(35) Adenine, N-hydroxy-
(36) Adriamycin   Suspected carcinogen
(37) Alanine, N-((5-chlori-8-hydroxy-
     3-methyl-1-oxo-7-isochromanyl)
     carbonyl)-3-phenyl-, (-)-   Suspected carcinogen
(38) Alloxan
(39) Ammonium, (2-chloroethyl) trim-
     ethyl-, chloride   Suspected carcinogen
(40) Ammonium, hecadecyltrimethyl-,
     bromide
(41) Anagyrine
(42) 5-alpha-Androstan-17-one, 3-alpha-
     hydroxy-
(43) Androst-4-ene-3, 17-dione   Suspected carcinogen
(44) Androst-4-en-3-one, 9-fluoro-11-beta,
     17-beta-dihydroxy-17-methyl-
(45) Androst-4-en-3-one, 17-beta-
     hydroxy-17-methyl-   Suspected carcinogen
(46) Androst-4-en-3-one, 17-beta-
     hydroxy-17-methyl- with testoster-
     one, propionate
(47) Angiotonin
(48) Aniline, N, N-dimethyl-p-((p-
     chlorophenyl)azo)-   Suspected carcinogen
(49) Aniline, N, N-dimethyl-p-(3-
     fluorophenylazo)-   Suspected carcinogen
(50) Aniline, N, N-dimethyl-p-phenylazo-   Category I carcinogen

TERATOGENIC SUBSTANCES   NOTE

(51) Aniline, N-ethyl-N-nitroso-
(52) Aniline, N-methyl-N-nitroso   Category I carcinogen
(53) Aniline, N-methyl-p-(phenylazo)-   Category I carcinogen
(54) Antipyrine, 4-(dimethylamino)-
(55) Antipyrine, 4-(dimethylamino)-
     molecular complex with 5, 5-
     diethylbarbituric acid (2:1)
(56) Arsenic   Category I carcinogen
(57) Arsenic acid, disodium salt,
     heptahydrate
(58) Arsenic acid, sodium salt   Suspected carcinogen
(59) Arsenious acid, monosodium salt   Suspected carcinogen
(60) Aspartic acid, N-phthaloyl-L-
(61) Azetidine-2-caroxylic acid, L-
(62) Azirino (2', 3': 3, 4) pyrrolo (1,2-a)
     indole-4, 7-dione, 6-amino-1, 1a, 2,
     8, 8a, 8b-hexahydro-8-(hydroxy
     methyl)-8a-methoxy-5-methyl-,
     carbamate (ester)   Suspected carcinogen
(63) Barbituric acid, 5, 5-diethyl-,
     sodium salt
(64) Barbituric acid, 5-ethyl-1-methyl-
     5-phenyl-
(65) Barbituric acid, 5-ethyl-5-phenyl-
(66) Barbituric acid, 5-ethyl-5-phenyl-,
     sodium salt   Category I carcinogen
(67) Benzanilide, 2-(2-(diethylamino)
     ethoxy)-
(68) Benzanilide, 2-(2-(diethylamino)
     ethoxy)-5-bromo-
(69) Benzanilide, 2-(2-(diethylamino)
     ethoxy)-5-chloro-
(70) Benzanilide, 2-(2-(diethylamino)
     ethoxy)-5-methyl-
(71) Benzanilide, 2-methyl-
(72) Benz (a) anthracene, 7, 12-dimethyl- Category I carcinogen

TERATOGENIC SUBSTANCES   *NOTE*

(73) Benz (a) anthracene-7-methanol,12-
    methyl-   Suspected carcinogen
(74) Benzene   Category I carcinogen
(75) m-Benzenedisulfonamide, 4, 5-
    dichloro-
(76) Benzene, hexachloro-   Suspected carcinogen
(77) Benzene, pentachloro-
(78) Benzene, pentachloronitro-   Suspected carcinogen
(79) Benzenesulfonamide, 4-chloro-N-
    ((cyclohexylcarbonyl)amino)-
(80) Benzenesulfonamide, N, N-diethyl-
(81) 2-Benzimidazolecarbamic acid, 1-
    butylcarbamoyl)-, methyl ester
(82) 2-Benzimidazolecarbamic acid, 5-
    butyl-, methyl ester
(83) 3H-1, 4-Benzodiazepine, 7-chloro-
    2-methylamino-5-phenyl-, 4-oxide,
    monohydrochloride
(84) 2H-1, 4-Benzodiazepin-2-one, 7-
    chloro-1, 3-dihydro-1-methyl-5-
    phenyl-
(85) 2H-1, 4-Benzodiazepin-2-one, 7-
    chloro-1, 3, -dihydro-5-phenyl-
(86) 2H-1, 4-Benzodiazepin-2-one,
    5-(o-chlorophenyl)-1, 3-dihydro-
    7-nitro-
(87) Benzoic acid, 2-hydroxy-, mono-
    sodium salt mixed with 3, 7-dihydro-
    3, 7-dimethyl-1H-purine-2, 6-dione
    sodium salt
(88) Benzoic acid, 3, 4, 5-trimethoxy-,
    2-(4-(3-(2-chloro-phenothiazin-10-
    yl)propyl)-1-piperazinyl) ethyl ester
(89) Benzo(a)pyrene   Category I carcinogen
(90) 2-Benzothiazolesulfonamide,
    6-ethoxy-

TERATOGENIC SUBSTANCES	NOTE
(91) Benzyl alcohol, alpha-(amino-methyl)-3, 4-dihydroxy-, (-)-	
(92) Benzyl alcohol, 3, 4-dihydroxy-alpha-((methylamino) methyl)-, (-)-	
(93) Biguanide, 1, 1-dimethyl-	
(94) Biphenyl, octabromo-	
(95) 2, 2'-Bipyridine	Suspected carcinogen
(96) 4, 4'-Bipyridinium, 1, 1'-dimethyl-, dichloride	
(97) Biurea, 1-methyl-6-(1-methylallyl)-2, 5-dithio-	
(98) Bleomycin	
(99) Bradykinin	
(100) Bredinin	
(101) 1, 4-Butanediol dimethylsulfonate	Suspected carcinogen
(102) 2-Butanone	Suspected carcinogen
(103) Butyric acid, 2-amino-4-(ethylthio)-, DL-	Category I carcinogen
(104) Butyric acid, 4-(5-bis(2-chloroethyl) amino-1-methyl-(1H)-benzimidazol-2-yl)-, hydrochloride	
(105) Butyric acid, 4-(p-bis(2-chloroethyl) aminophenyl)-	Category I carcinogen
(106) Butyric acid, 4-(2, 4, 5-trichloro-phenoxy)-	
(107) Butyrophenone, 4-(4-(p-chloro-phenyl)-4-hydroxy-piperidino)-4'-fluoro-	
(108) Butyrophenone, 4'-fluoro-4-(4-hydroxy-4-(alpha, alpha, alpha-tri-fluoro-m-tolyl)piperidino)-	
(109) Cadmium	Category I carcinogen
(110) Cadmium chloride	Category I carcinogen
(111) Cadmium sulfate (1:1)	Category I carcinogen
(112) Caffeine	
(113) Calcium fluoride	
(114) Cannabis	

TERATOGENIC SUBSTANCES	NOTE
(115) Carbamic acid, ethyl ester	Category I carcinogen
(116) Carbamic acid, ethylnitroso-, ethyl ester	
(117) Carbamic acid, hydroxy-, ethyl ester	Suspected carcinogen
(118) Carbamic acid, 2-hydroxethyl ester	
(119) Carbamic acid, methyl-, ethyl ester	Suspected carcinogen
(120) Carbamic acid, methyl-, 1-napthyl ester	Suspected carcinogen
(121) Carbamic acid, N-methyl-N-nitroso-, ethyl ester	Category I carcinogen
(122) Carbamic acid, propyl ester	Suspected carcinogen
(123) Carbanilic acid, p-carboxy-, 4-bis (2-chloroethylamino)phenyl ester	
(124) Carbon dioxide	
(125) Carbonic acid, diethyl ester	Suspected carcinogen
(126) Carbon monoxide	
(127) Carbon tetrachloride	Category I carcinogen
(128) Carmine, lithium salt	
(129) alpha-Chaconine	
(130) Chloroform	Category I carcinogen
(131) Cholanthrene, 3-methyl	Category I carcinogen
(132) Cholesterol	Suspected carcinogen
(133) Chondroitin sulfate	
(134) Chromium (VI) oxide (1:3)	Category I carcinogen
(135) Chromomycin A3	
(136) Colchicine	Suspected carcinogen
(137) Colchicine, N-deacetyl-N-methyl-	Suspected carcinogen
(138) Corticosterone	
(139) Corticosterone, 21-acetate	
(140) Corticotropin	
(141) Cortisol	
(142) Cortisol, 21-acetate	
(143) Cortisol, succinate, sodium salt	
(144) Cortisone	
(145) Cortisone 21-acetate	
(146) Cottonseed oil (deodorized winterized)	

TERATOGENIC SUBSTANCES   NOTE

(147) Coumarin, 3-(alpha-acetonylbenzyl)-
       4-hydroxy-
(148) 1, 4-Cyclohexanebis (methylamine),
       N, N′-bis(2-chlorobenzyl)-, dihydro-
       chloride, (E)-
(149) Cyclohexene-1, 2-dicarboximide
(150) 4-Cyclohexene-1, 2-dicarboximide,
       N-((1, 1, 2, 2-tetrachloroethyl)thio)-   Suspected carcinogen
(151) 4-Cyclohexene-1, 2-dicarboximide,
       N-(trichloromethyl)thio-   Suspected carcinogen
(152) 1H-Cyclonona(1, 2-c:5, 6-c′)difuran-
       1, 3, 6, 8 (4H)-tetrone, 10-((3, 6-
       dihydro-6-oxo-2H-pyran-2-yl)
       hydroxymethyl)-5, 9, 10, 11-tetra-
       hydro-4-hydroxy-5-(1-hydroxy-
       heptyl)-
(153) Cyclopamine
(154) Cyclopenta(c)furo(3′, 2′:4, 5)furo(2,
       3-h)(1)benzopyran-1, 11-dione, 2, 3,
       6a, 9a-tetrahydro-4-methoxy-   Category I carcinogen
(155) Cycloposine
(156) Cyclopropanealanine, 2-methylene-
(157) 3′H-Cyclopropa (1, 2) pregna-1,
       4, 6-triene-3, 20-dione, 6-chloro-1-
       beta, 2-beta-dihydro-17-hydroxy-,
       acetate
(158) Cyclosiloxane, methyl phenyl-
(159) Cypromate
(160) Cytidine, 5-bromo-2′-deoxy-
(161) Cytidine, 2′-deoxy-5-fluoro-
(162) Cytidine, 2′-deoxy-5-fluoro-N-
       methyl-
(163) Cytochalasin D
(164) Cytosine, 1-beta-D-arabinofurano-
       syl-   Suspected carcinogen
(165) Cytosine, 1-beta-D-arabinofurano-
       syl-2, 2′-anhydro-, hydrochloride

TERATOGENIC SUBSTANCES   NOTE

(166) Cytosine, 1-beta-D-arabinofurano-
       syl-5-fluoro-
(167) Cytosine, 5-fluoro-
(168) Daunomycin   Category I carcinogen
(169) 5H-Dibenz(b, f)azepine-5-carboxa-
       mide
(170) 5H-Dibenz(b, f)azepine, 5-(3-(dime-
       thylamino)propyl)-10, 11-dihydro-
(171) 5H-Dibenz(b, f)azepine, 5-(3-(dime-
       thylamino)propyl)-10, 11-dihydro-,
       monohydrochloride
(172) 5H-Dibenz(b, f)azepine, 5-(3-(dime-
       thylamino)propyl)-10, 11-dihydro-,
       5-oxide, monohydrochloride
(173) Dibenzo-p-dioxin, hexchloro-   Suspected carcinogen
(174) Dibenzo-p-dioxin, 2,3,7,8-tetrachloro- Suspected carcinogen
(175) 6H-Dibenzo(b, d)pyran-1-ol, 6a, 7, 8,
       10a-tetrahydro-6, 6, 9-trimethyl-3-
       pentyl-
(176) Diethylamine, 2, 2'-dichloro-,
       hydrochloride
(177) Diethylamine, 2, 2'-dichloro-N-
       methyl-   Category I carcinogen
(178) Diethylamine, 2, 2'-dichloro-N-
       methyl, hydrochloride   Category I carcinogen
(179) Diethylamine, N-nitroso-   Category I carcinogen
(180) Dimethanesulfonic acid, trimethy-
       lene ester
(181) 1, 4:5, 8-Dimethanonaphthalene, 1,
       2, 3, 4, 10, 10-hexachloro-6, 7-epoxy-
       1, 4, 4a, 5, 6, 7, 8, 8a-octahydro-,
       endo, endo-   Suspected carcinogen
(182) 1, 4:5, 8-Dimethanonapthalene, 1, 2,
       3, 4, 10, 10-hexachloro-6, 7-epoxy-1, 4,
       4a, 5, 6, 7, 8, 8a-octahydro-, endo, exo- Suspected carcinogen
(183) 1, 4:5, 8-Dimethanonapthalene, 1,
       2, 3, 4, 10, 10-hexachloro-1, 4, 4a, 5,

TERATOGENIC SUBSTANCES   *NOTE*

	8, 8a-hexahydro-, endo, exo-	Suspected carcinogen
(184)	Diphenylamine	Suspected carcinogen
(185)	Disulfide, bis(dimethylthiocarbamoyl)	
(186)	Dithane M-45	
(187)	Duazomycin	
(188)	Dye C	
(189)	2-alpha, 3-alpha-Epithio-5-alpha-androstan-17-beta-ol	
(190)	Ergoline-8-beta-carboxamide, 2-bromo-9, 10-didehydro-N, N-diethyl-6-methyl-	
(191)	Ergoline-8-beta-carboxamide, 9, 10-didehydro-N, N-diethyl-6-methyl	
(192)	Ergoline-8-methanol, 8, 9-didehydro-6-methyl-	
(193)	Ergotamine tartrate	
(194)	Estradiol	Category I carcinogen
(195)	Estradiol, 3-benzoate	Category I carcinogen
(196)	Estr-4-en-17-beta-ol, 17-allyl-	
(197)	Estrone	Category I carcinogen
(198)	Ethane, azo-	Category I carcinogen
(199)	Ethane, azoxy	Category I carcinogen
(200)	Ethane, 2-bromo-2-chloro-1, 1, 1-trifluoro-	
(201)	Ethane, 1, 1-dichloro	Suspected carcinogen
(202)	9, 10-Ethanoanthracene-9-(10H)-methylamine, N-methyl-, hydrochloride	
(203)	Ethanol, 2-(2-(4-(p-chloro-alpha-phenylbenzyl)-1-piperazinyl) ethoxy)-	
(204)	Ethanol, 2-(2-(4-(p-chloro-alpha-phenylbenzyl)-1-piperazinyl) ethoxy)-, monohydrochloride	
(205)	Ethanol, 2-(p-chlorophenyl)-1-(p-	

TERATOGENIC SUBSTANCES   NOTE

     (2-(diethylamino) ethoxy)phenyl)-
     1-p-tolyl-
(206) Ethanol, 1-(p-(2-(diethylamino)
     ethoxy)phenyl)-2-(p-methoxy-
     phenyl)-1-phenyl-
(207) Ether, bis(pentabromophenyl)
(208) Ether, 2, 4-dichlorophenyl
     p-nitrophenyl
(209) Ethyl alcohol   Suspected carcinogen
(210) Ethylamine, N, N-dimethyl-2-((o-
     methyl-alpha-phenylbenzyl)oxy)-,
     hydrochloride
(211) Ethylenemethanesulfonate
(212) Firemaster BP-6
(213) Formamide
(214) Formamide, N-methyl
(215) Formhydroxamic acid
(216) 2-Furaldehyde, 5-nitro-, semicar-
     bazone   Suspected carcinogen
(217) Galactose, D-
(218) Glutamic acid, N-(p-(((2, 4-diamino-
     6-pteridinyl)methyl)amino)
     benzoyl)-, L-   Suspected carcinogen
(219) Glutamic acid, N-(p-(((2, 4-diamino-
     6-pteridinyl)methyl)methylamino)
     benzoyl)-, L-   Suspected carcinogen
(220) Glutamic acid, N-(p-(((2, 4-diamino-
     6-pteridinyl)methyl)methylamino)
     benzoyl)-, sodium salt
(221) Glutamic acid, monosodium salt,
     L-(+)-
(222) Glutaramic acid, 4-phthalimido-,
     methyl ester, DL
(223) Glutaramic acid, 4-phthalyl-
(224) Glutarimide, N-methyl-2-phthali-
     mido-
(225) Glycine, N, N-bis (2-(bis(carboxy-

TERATOGENIC SUBSTANCES   *NOTE*

    methyl)amino)ethyl)-, calcium salt
(226) Glycine, N-formyl-N-hydroxy-
(227) Glycinonitrile
(228) Glycinonitrile, sulfate (2:1)
(229) Heliotrine   Suspected carcinogen
(230) 3-Heptanone, 6-(dimethylamino)-
      4, 4-diphenyl-
(231) Hexanoic acid, 6-amino-
(232) D-arabino-hexose, 2-deoxy-
(233) Hydantoin, 5, 5-diphenyl-   Suspected carcinogen
(234) Hydantoin, 5, 5-diphenyl-, mono-
      sodium salt   Suspected carcinogen
(235) Hydantoin, 1-((5-nitrofurfurylidene)
      amino)-
(236) Hydrazine, 1-(p-allophanoylben-
      zyl)-2-methyl, hydrobromide
(237) Hydrazine, 2-benzyl-1-methyl-   Suspected carcinogen
(238) Hydrazine, 1-(o-chlorophenethyl)-,
      hydrogen sulfate (1:2)
(239) Hydrazine, 1, 2-diethyl-, dihydro-
      chloride   Suspected carcinogen
(240) Hydrazine, methyl-   Suspected carcinogen
(241) Hydrouracil, 5-bromo-1-(2-deoxy-
      beta-D-ribofuranosyl)-5-fluoro-6-
      methoxy-
(242) Imidazole-4-carboxamide, 5-(3, 3-
      dimethyl-1-triazeno)-, citrate
(243) 2-Imidazolidinethione   Suspected carcinogen
(244) 2-Imidazolidinethione, 4-methyl-
(245) 2-Imidazolidinethione mixed with
      sodium nitrite
(246) 1, 3-Indandione
(247) 1, 3-Indandione, 2-(3-ethoxy-1-in-
      danylidene)-
(248) 1, 3-Indandione, 2-methyl-
(249) 1, 3-Indandione, 2-(3-oxo-1-indany-

TERATOGENIC SUBSTANCES   *NOTE*

	lidene)-	
(250)	Indium nitrate	
(251)	1H-Indole-3-acetic acid	
(252)	Indole, 3-(2-aminopropyl)-	
(253)	Indol-5-ol, 3-(2-aminoethyl)-	
(254)	Indol-5-ol, 3-(2-aminoethyl)-, compd. with creatinine sulfate	
(255)	Insulin, ultra lente	Suspected carcinogen
(256)	Isonicotinamide, 2-ethylthio-	
(257)	Isonicotinic acid hydrazide	Category I carcinogen
(258)	Lactose	Suspected carcinogen
(259)	Lead chloride	
(260)	Lead(II) nitrate (1:2)	
(261)	Leucine, L-	
(262)	Leurocristine	Suspected carcinogen
(263)	Leurocristine sulfate (1:1)	
(264)	Linoleic acid (oxidized)	
(265)	Lithium	
(266)	Lithium carbonate (2:1)	
(267)	Lithium chloride	
(268)	Lupinus	
(269)	Maleimide	
(270)	Maleimide, dibromo-	
(271)	Maleimide, dibromo-N-methyl-	
(272)	Maleimide, dichloro-	
(273)	Maleimide, 2, 3-dichloro-N-ethyl-	
(274)	Maleimide, 2, 3-dichloro-N-methyl-	
(275)	Manganese, (ethylenebis(dithiocarbamato))-	Suspected carcinogen
(276)	Manganese, (ethylenebis(dithiocarbamato)- and zinc acetate (50:1)	
(277)	Mannitol, 1, 6-dibromo-1, 6-dideoxy-, D-	Suspected carcinogen
(278)	Maytansine	
(279)	Mercury, (acetato) phenyl-	Suspected carcinogen
(280)	Mercury, chloromethyl-	

TERATOGENIC SUBSTANCES   *NOTE*

(281) Mercury, (3-cyanoguanidino)
        methyl-
(282) Methacrylic acid, butyl ester
(283) Methacrylic acid, ethyl ester
(284) Methacrylic acid, isobutyl ester
(285) Methacrylic acid, isodecyl ester
(286) Methacrylic acid, methyl ester   Suspected carcinogen
(287) Methanediol, dimethanesulfonate
(288) Methanesulfonanilide, 2'-hydroxy-
        5'-(1-hydroxy-2-(isopropylamino)
        ethyl)-, monohydrochloride   Suspected carcinogen
(289) Methanesulfonic acid, (antipy-
        rinylmethylamino)-, monosodium
        salt
(290) Methanesulfonic acid, ethyl ester   Category I carcinogen
(291) Methanesulfonic acid, isopropyl
        ester
(292) Methanol, (methyl-ONN-azoxy)-   Category I carcinogen
(293) Mehanol, (methyl-ONN-azoxy)-,
        acetate (ester)   Category I carcinogen
(294) 1, 3, 4-Metheno-1H-cyclobuta(cd)
        pentalene, 1, 1a, 2, 2, 3, 3a, 4, 5, 5,
        5a, 5b, 6-dodecachlorooctahydro-   Category I carcinogen
(295) Methyl sulfoxide
(296) Morpholine, 3-methyl-2-phenyl-,
        hydrochloride
(297) 2-Naphthacenecarboxamide, 4-
        (dimethylamino)-1, 4, 4a, 5, 5a, 6,
        11, 12a-octahydro-3, 5, 6, 10, 12,
        12a-hexahydroxy-6-methyl-1, 11-
        dioxo-
(298) 2-Naphthacenecarboxamide, 4-
        (dimethylamino)-1, 4, 4a, 5, 5a, 6,
        11, 12a-octahydro-3, 6, 10, 12, 12a-
        pentahydroxy-6-methyl-9-(morpho-
        linomethyl)-1, 11-dioxo-

TERATOGENIC SUBSTANCES   NOTE

(299) 3, 6-Naphthalenedisulfonic acid, 8-
       amino-7-hydroxy-, sodium salt
(300) 2, 7-Naphthalenedisulfonic acid, 3,
       3'-((4, 4'-biphenylylene) bis(azo))-
       bis(5-amino-4-hydroxy)-, tetraso-
       dium salt   Suspected carcinogen
(301) 2, 7-Naphthalenedisulfonic acid, 3,
       3'((3, 3'-dichloro-4, 4'-biphenyly-
       lene)-bis(azo))bis(5-amino-4-
       hydroxy)-, tetrasodium salt
(302) 2, 7-Naphthalenedisulfonic acid, 3,
       3'-((3,3'-dimethoxy-4, 4'-biphenyl-
       ylene)bis(azo)bis(5-amino-4-
       hydroxy)-,tetrasodium salt
(303) 6, 8 Naphthalcnedisulfonic acid, 3,
       3'-((3, 3'-dimethoxy-4, 4'-bipheny-
       lene)bis(azo)bis)(5-amino-4-
       hydroxy)-, tetrasodium salt
(304) 1, 3-Naphthalenedisulfonic acid, 6,
       6'-((3, 3'-dimethyl-4, 4'-biphenyly-
       lene)bis(azo))bis(4-amino-5-hydroxy)-,
       tetrasodium salt
(305) 2, 7-Naphthalenedisulfonic acid, 3,
       3'-((3, 3'-dimethyl-4, 4'-biphenyly-
       lene)-bis(azo))bis(5-amino-4-
       hydroxy)-, tetrasodium salt   Category I carcinogen
(306) 2, 7-Naphthalenedisulfonic acid,
       3-hydroxy-4-((4-sulfo-1-naphthyl)
       azo)-, trisodium salt   Suspected carcinogen
(307) 2-Naphthalenesulfonic acid, 5-
       amino-, sodium salt
(308) Naphthalenesulfonic acid, 3, 3'-
       ((4, 4'-biphenylenebis(azo))bis(4-
       amino)-, disodium salt
(309) 2-Naphthoic acid, 4, 4'-methylenebis
       (3-hydroxy)-, ester with 2-(2-(4-(p-

    chloro-alpha-phenylbenzyl)-1-
    piperazinyl)-ethoxy)ethanol
(310) Nicotine   Suspected carcinogen
(311) Nitrogen oxide
(312) 5-Norbornene-2, 3-dimethanol, 1, 4,
    5, 6, 7, 7-hexchloro-, cyclic sulfite   Suspected carcinogen
(313) Norleucine, 6-diazo-5-oxo-
(314) 19-nor-17-alpha-Pregn-5(10)-en-20-
    yn-3-alpha-17-beta-diol
(315) 19-nor-17-alpha-Pregn-5(10)-en-20-
    yn-3-beta-17-beta-diol
(316) 19-nor-17-alpha-Pregn-5(10)-en-20-
    yn-3-one, 17-hydroxy-   Category I carcinogen
(317) 19-nor-17-alpha-Pregn-4-en-20-yn
    3-one, 17-hydroxy-, heptanate
(318) 19-nor-17-alpha-Pregn-4-en-20-yn-
    3-one, 17-hydroxy-mixed with 3-
    methoxy-19-nor-17-alpha-pregna-1,
    3, 5(10)-trien-20-yn-17-ol
(319) Oxazaphosphorine, 2-(bis(2-chloro-
    ethyl)amino)tetrahydro-, cyclo-
    hexylamine salt   Suspected carcinogen
(320) 2H-1, 3, 2-Oxazaphosphorine, 2-
    (bis(2-chloroethyl)amino) tetra-
    hydro-, 2-oxide   Category I carcinogen
(321) 2, 4-Oxazolidinedione, 5, 5-dimethyl-
(322) 2, 4-Oxazolidinedione, 3, 5, 5-
    trimethyl
(323) Oxonic acid, potassium salt
(324) Penitrem A
(325) Phenethylamine, N, alpha-dimethyl-
(326) Phenethylamine, N, alpha-dimethyl-,
    hydrochloride, (-)-
(327) Phenethylamine, alpha-methyl-,
    sulfate (2:1), (+)-
(328) Phenethylamine, 3, 4, 5-trimethoxy-

TERATOGENIC SUBSTANCES   NOTE

(329) Phenol, 2-amino-4-arsenoso-,
       hydrochloride
(330) Phenol, 2-sec-butyl-4, 6-dinitro-   Suspected carcinogen
(331) Phenol, 2, 2'-methylenebis (3, 4, 6-
       trichloro)-   Suspected carcinogen
(332) Phenol, pentachloro-   Suspected carcinogen
(333) Phenothiazine, 2-chloro-10-(3-
       (dimethylamino)propyl)-
(334) Phenothiazine, 2-chloro-10-(3-
       (dimethylamino)propyl),-monohy-
       drochloride
(335) Phenothiazine, 2-chloro-10-(3-(4-
       methyl-1-piperazinyl)propyl)-
(336) p-Phenylenediamine, N, N-bis(2-
       chloroethyl)-
(337) Phosphine oxide, bis (1-aziridinyl)
       methyl-
(338) Phosphine oxide, tris(1-(2-methyl)
       aziridinyl)-
(339) Phosphine sulfide, tris(1-aziridinyl)-   Suspected carcinogen
(340) Phosphonic acid, (1-hydroxy-2, 2, 2-
       trichloroethyl)-, diethyl ester
(341) Phosphonic acid, (2, 2, 2-trichloro-
       1-hydroxyethyl)-,dimethyl ester   Suspected carcinogen
(342) Phosphoramidic acid, N, N-bis(2-
       chloroethyl)-O-(3-aminopropyl)-,
       inner salt
(343) Phosphoric acid, 2, 2-dichlorovinyl
       dimethyl ester   Suspected carcinogen
(344) Phosphorodiamidic acid, N, N-bis
       (2-chloroethyl)-,cyclohexylamine salt
(345) Phosphorodithioic acid, S-(2-chloro-
       1-(1, 3-dihydro-1, 3-dioxo-2H-isoin-
       dol-2-yl)ethyl)O, O-diethyl ester
(346) Phosphorodithioic acid, O,
       O-dimethyl

ester, S-ester with N-(mercapto-methyl)phthalimide	Suspected carcinogen
(347) Phosphorothioic acid, O, O-diethyl O-(2-(ethylthio)ethyl) ester, mixed with O, O-diethyl S-(2-(ethylthio) ethyl) ester (7:3)	
(348) Phosphorothioic acid, O, O-diethyl O-(2-isopropyl-6-methyl-4-pyrimidinyl) ester	Suspected carcinogen
(349) Phosphorothioic acid, O, O-diethyl O-(p-nitrophenyl) ester	Suspected carcinogen
(350) Phosphorothioic acid, O, O-dimethyl-, O-(4-methylthio)-m-tolyl) ester	Suspected carcinogen
(351) Phosphorothioic acid, O, O-di-methyl-, O-(p-nitrophenyl) ester	Suspected carcinogen
(352) Phthalic acid, bis(2-ethylhexyl) ester	Suspected carcinogen
(353) Phthalic acid, butoxycarbonyl-methyl butyl ester	Suspected carcinogen
(354) Phthalic acid, dibutyl ester	Suspected carcinogen
(355) Phthalic acid, diethyl ester	Suspected carcinogen
(356) Phthalic acid, diisobutyl ester	Suspected carcinogen
(357) Phthalic acid, di(methoxyethyl) ester	Suspected carcinogen
(358) Phthalic acid, dimethyl ester	Suspected carcinogen
(359) Phthalic acid, dioctyl ester	Suspected carcinogen
(360) Phthalimide	Suspected carcinogen
(361) Phthalimide, N-(2, 6-dioxo-3-piperidyl)-	
(362) Phthalimide, (-)-N-(2, 6-dioxo-3-piperidyl)-	
(363) Phthalimide, (+)-N-(2,6,-dioxo-3-piperidyl)-	
(364) Phthalimide, (+-)-N-(2, 6-dioxo-3-piperidyl)-	
(365) Phthalimide, N-((trichloromethyl) thio)-	

TERATOGENIC SUBSTANCES   *NOTE*

(366) Phthalimidine, 2-(2, 6-dioxopiper-
       iden-3-yl)-
(367) Picolinic acid, 5-amino-6-(7-amino-
       5, 8-dihydro-6-methoxy-5, 8-dioxo-
       2-quinolyl)-4-(2-hydroxy-3, 4-dime-
       thoxyphenyl)-3-methyl-
(368) Piperazine, 1-(p-tert-butylbenzyl)-
       4-(p-chloro-alpha-phenylbenzyl)-,
       dihydrochloride
(369) Piperazine, 1-(p-chloro-alpha-
       phenylbenzyl)-4-methyl-
(370) Piperazine, 1-(p-chloro-alpha-
       phenylbenzyl)-4-methyl-,
       monohydrochloride
(371) 2, 6-Piperazinedione, 4, 4'-propyl-
       enedi-, (+-)-
(372) 1-Piperazineethanol, 4-(3-(2-chloro-
       phenothiazin-10-yl) propyl)-,
       monohydrochloride
(373) Piperidine, 2-propyl-
(374) Polychlorinated triphenyl
(375) Potato, green parts
(376) Pregna-4, 6-diene-3, 20-dione, 6-
       chloro-17-hydroxy-, acetate   Suspected carcinogen
(377) Pregna-1, 4-diene-3, 20-dione, 6, 9-
       difluoro-11, 12-dihydroxy-16, 17-((1-
       methylethylidene)bis(oxy))-, (6-
       alpha, 11-beta, 16-alpha)-
(378) Pregna-1, 4-diene-3, 20-dione, 9-
       fluoro-11-beta, 16-alpha, 17, 21-
       tetrahydroxy-
(379) Pregna-1, 4-diene-3, 20-dione, 9-
       fluoro-11-beta, 16-alpha, 17, 21-
       tetrahydroxy-, cyclic 16, 17-acetal
       with acetone
(380) Pregna-1, 4-diene-3, 20-dione, 9-
       fluoro-11-beta, 17, 21-trihydroxy-

16-alpha-methyl-
(381) Pregna-1, 4-diene-3, 20-dione, 9-
fluoro-11-beta, 17, 21-trihydroxy-
16-beta-methyl-
(382) Pregna-1, 4-diene-3, 20-dione, 9-
fluoro-11-beta, 17, 21-trihydroxy-
16-alpha-methyl-, acetate-
(383) 9-beta, 10-alpha-Pregna-4, 6-diene-
3, 20-dione and 17-alpha-hydroxy-
pregn-4-ene-3, 20-dione (9:10)
(384) Pregna-1, 4-diene-3, 20-dione, 6-
alpha-methyl-11-beta-17, 21-trihy-
droxy-
(385) Pregna-1, 4-diene-3, 20-dione, 11-
beta, 17, 21-trihydroxy-
(386) (6-alpha)-Pregn-4-ene-3, 20-dione,
17-(acetyloxy)-6-methyl-
(387) Progesterone   Category I carcinogen
(388) 1, 2-Propanediol, diacetate
(389) 1, 3-Propanediol, 2-methyl-2-
propyl-, dicarbamate
(390) 1-propanol, 2, 3-dimercapto-
(391) 2-Propanone, 1, 1, 1, 3, 3, 3-hexa-
fluoro-
(392) Propionic acid, 2-(2, 4, 5-trichloro-
phenoxy)-
(393) Propionitrile, 3-amino-
(394) Propionitrile, 3-amino-, fumarate
(2:1)
(395) Prosta-5, 13-dien-1-oic acid, (5Z, 11-
alpha, 13E, 15S)-11, 15-dihydroxy-
9-oxo-
(396) Prostaglandin A1
(397) Purine, 2-amino-6-((1-methyl-4-
nitroimidazol-5-yl)thio)-
(398) Purine, 6-chloro-

TERATOGENIC SUBSTANCES   *NOTE*

(399) Purine, 6-thiol   Suspected carcinogen

(400) 9H-Purine-6-thiol, 2-amino-9-beta-
D-ribofuranosyl-

(401) 9H-purine-6-thiol, 9-butyl-

(402) 9H-purine-6-thiol, 9-ethyl-

(403) Purin-6-thiol, 3-N-oxide

(404) 9H-Purine-6-thiol, 9-ribofuranosyl-

(405) Purine-6(1H)-thione, 2-amino-

(406) 3, 5-Pyrazolidinedione, 4-butyl-1, 2-
diphenyl-

(407) 3-Pyridinecarboxamide, 6-amino-

(408) 2, 3-Pyridinecarboximide

(409) 3, 4-Pyridinecarboximide

(410) Pyridine-1-oxide, 2, 2'-dithiobis-,
magnesium sulfate, trihydrate

(411) 1 (4H)-Pyridinepropionic acid,
alpha-amino-3-hydroxy-4-oxo-

(412) Pyridinium, 1-((2-carboxy-8-oxo-7-
(2-(2-thienyl)acetamido)-5-thia-1-
azabicyclo (4.2.0) oct-2-en-3-yl)
methyl)-, hydroxide, inner salt

(413) 4-Pyrimidinecarboxylic acid, 1, 2,
3, 6-tetrahydro-2, 6-dioxo-5-fluoro-

(414) 2, 4-Pyrimidinediamine, 5-(p-
chlorophenyl)-6-ethyl-

(415) 4, 6 (1H, 5H)-Pyrimidinedione, 5-
ethyldihydro-5-phenyl-

(416) Pyrrolidine, 1-(2-(p-(alpha-(p-
methoxyphenyl)-beta-nitrostryryl)
phenoxy)ethyl)-monocitrate

(417) 5H-Pyrrolo (3, 4-b)pyrazine, 5, 7
(6H)-dioxo-

(418) 5H-Pyrrolo (3, 4-d) pyrimidine, 5,
7(6H)-dioxo-

(419) 4 (3H)-Quinazolinone, 2-methyl-3-
o-tolyl-

TERATOGENIC SUBSTANCES *NOTE*

(420) Quinine

(421) Quinine, sulfate

(422) Quinoline, 7-chloro-4-((4-(diethyl-amino)-1-methylbutyl)amino)-

(423) Resorcylic acid, 6-(10-hydroxy-6-oxo-1-undecenyl)-, mu-lactone, trans-

(424) Retinoic acid, all-trans-

(425) Retinoic acid, all-trans-, sodium salt

(426) Retinol, all trans-

(427) Retinol, acetate

(428) Retinol, all-trans-, palmitate

(429) Rifomycin SV, 3-(N-(4-methyl-1-piperazinyl)formidoyl)-

(430) Rubidomycin

(431) Salicyclic acid

(432) Salicylic acid, acetate

(433) Salicylic acid, 4-amino-, sodium salt

(434) Salicylic acid, methyl ester

(435) Salicylic acid, monosodium salt

(436) Sarkomycin — Suspected carcinogen

(437) Semicarbazide, monohydrochloride — Suspected carcinogen

(438) Serine, diazoacetate (ester) — Suspected carcinogen

(439) Sodium chloride

(440) Sodium fluoride

(441) Solanid-5-ene, 3-beta-((O-6-deoxy-alpha-L-mannopyranosyl-O(beta-D-glucopyranosyl-L-beta-D-galacto-pyranosyl)oxy)-

(442) Solasod-5-en-3-beta-ol

(443) Spiro(9H-benzo(a)fluorene-9-2' (3'H)-furo(3, 2-b)-pyridin)-11(1H)-O-NE, 2, 3, 3'a, 4, 4', 5', 6, 6', 6a, 6b, 7, 7', 7'a, 8, 11a, 11b-hexadecahydro-3-hydroxy-3', 6', 10, 11b-tetramethyl-

TERATOGENIC SUBSTANCES   NOTE

(444) Spiro(benzofuran-2(3H), 1'-(2)cyclo-
      hexene-3, 4'-dione, 7-chloro-2', 4,
      6-trimethoxy-6'-beta-methyl-   Category I carcinogen
(445) 4, 4'-Stilbenediol, alpha, alpha'-
      diethyl   Category I carcinogen
(446) Streptomycin
(447) Styrene, methyl-
(448) Succinimide, 2-ethyl-2-methyl-
(449) Sulfonic acid, alpha-alkene-
(450) Sweet pea seeds
(451) Tellurium
(452) Testosterone   Category I carcinogen
(453) Testosterone, propionate   Category I carcinogen
(454) Theobromine
(455) Theophylline
(456) Theophylline, 8-benzyl-7-(2-(ethyl
      (2-hydroxyethyl)amino)ethyl)-
(457) Theophylline, 8-benzyl-7-(1'-
      morpholino-2'-amino)ethyl-,
      hydrochloride
(458) Theophylline, compd. with ethyl-
      enediamine (2:1)
(459) 5-Thia,1-azabicyclo (4.2.0) oct-2-
      ene-2-carboxylic acid, 6R-(3-
      (acetyloxy)methyl)-8-oxo-7-((2-
      thienylacetyl)amino)-
(460) 1, 3, 4-Thiadiazole, 2-amino-
(461) 1, 3, 4-Thiadiazole, 2-amino-,
      hydrochloride
(462) 1, 3, 4-Thiadiazole, 2-ethylamino-,
      2'-methylenebis(imino)-
(463) 1, 3, 4-Thiadiazole, 2, 2'-methyl-
      enebis(imino)-
(464) 1, 3, 4-Thiadiazole-5-sulfonamide,
      2-amino-
(465) 1, 3, 4-Thiadiazole-5-sulfonamide,

TERATOGENIC SUBSTANCES   *NOTE*

2-(phenylsulfonylamino)-	
(466) 9H-Thioxanthen-9-one, 1-((2-(diethylamino)ethyl)amino)-4-(hydroxymethyl)-, monomethane-sulfonate (salt)	
(467) p-Toluamide, N-isopropyl-alpha-(2-methylhydrazino)-	Category I carcinogen
(468) Toluene-2, 5-diamine dihydro-chloride	
(469) p-Toluidine, alpha, alpha, alpha-trifluoro-2, 6-dinitro-N, N-dipropyl-	Suspected carcinogen
(470) Toxaphene	Suspected carcinogen
(471) 1, 3, 5, 2, 4, 6-Triazatriphosphorine, 2, 2, 4, 4, 6, 6-hexakis (1-aziridinyl)-2, 2, 4, 4, 6, 6-hexahydro-	Suspected carcinogen
(472) Triazene, 3, 3-dimethyl-1-phenyl-	Category I carcinogen
(473) Triazene, 3, 3-dimethyl-1-(m-pyridyl)-	Suspected carcinogen
(474) Triazene, 3-ethyl-3-methyl-1-pyridyl-	
(475) Triazene, 1-ethyl-3-phenyl	
(476) Triazene, 3-monomethyl-1-phenyl-	
(477) as-Triazine-3, 5(2H, 4H)-dione, 2-beta-D-ribofuranosyl-	
(478) as-Triazine-3, 5-(2H, 4H)-dione, 2-(2', 3', 5'-triacetyl-beta-D-ribofuranosyl)-	
(479) s-Triazine, 2, 4, 6-tris (1-aziridinyl)-	Suspected carcinogen
(480) as-Triazin-3(2H)-one, 5-amino-2-beta-D-ribofuranosyl-	
(481) 7H-v-Triazolo (4, 5-d)pyrimidin-7-one, 5-amino-1, 6-dihydro-	
(482) delta-9-Trichothecane, 4, 15-diacetoxy-12, 13-epoxy-3-hydroxy-9-(3-naphthylbutyryloxy)-	
(483) Triethylamine, 2-(p-(2-chloro-1, 2-diphenylvinyl)phenoxy)-	

TERATOGENIC SUBSTANCES   NOTE

(484) Triethylamine, 2-(p-(2-chloro-1, 2-
       diphenylvinyl)phenoxy)-, citrate
(485) Triethylamine, 2-(p-(1, 2, 3, 4-tetra-
       hydro-2-(p-chlorophenyl)naphthyl)
       phenoxy)-
(486) Triton WR-1339
(487) Uracil, 5-(bis(2-chloroethyl)amino)-   Category I carcinogen
(488) Uracil, 5-fluoro-   Suspected carcinogen
(489) Uracil, 6-methyl-2-thio-   Category I carcinogen
(490) Urea, 1, 3-bis(2-chloroethyl)-1-
       nitroso-
(491) Urea, 1-butyl-3-sulfanilyl-
(492) Urea, 1-butyl-3-(p-tolylsulfonyl)-   Suspected carcinogen
(493) Urea, 1-butyl-3-(p-tolylsulfonyl)-,
       sodium salt   Suspected carcinogen
(494) Urea, 1-(2-chloroethyl)-3-cyclohexyl-
       1-nitroso-
(495) Urea, 3-(p-chlorophenyl)-1-
       methoxy-1-methyl-
(496) Urea, 3-(p-chlorophenyl)-1-methyl-
       1-(1-methyl-2-propynyl)-
(497) Urea, 1-((p-chlorophenyl)sulfonyl)-
       3-propyl-   Suspected carcinogen
(498) Urea, 1-cyclohexyl-3-(4-methyl-
       metanilyl)-   Suspected carcinogen
(499) Urea, 1, 3-dimethyl-
(500) Urea, 1, 3-dimethyl-1-nitroso-   Suspected carcinogen
(501) Urea, 1-ethyl-1-nitroso-   Suspected carcinogen
(502) Urea, ethyl- and sodium nitrite (2:1)   Suspected carcinogen
(503) Urea, hydroxy-   Suspected carcinogen
(504) Urea, N-methyl-N-nitroso-   Suspected carcinogen
(505) Urea, N-nitroso-N-propyl-   Suspected carcinogen
(506) Urea, N-nitrosotrimethyl-
(507) Urea, 1, 1, 3, 3-tetramethyl-
(508) Urea, 1, 1, 3, 3-tetramethyl-2-thio-
(509) Urea, 1, 1, 3-trimethyl-

TERATOGENIC SUBSTANCES   NOTE

(510) Uridine, 5-bromo-2'-deoxy-
(511) Uridine, 5-chloro-2'-deoxy-
(512) Uridine, 2'-deoxy-5-fluoro-
(513) Uridine, 2'-deoxy-5-iodo-
(514) Uridine, 5-fluoro-
(515) Valeric acid, 2-propyl-, sodium salt
(516) Valine, 3-mercapto-, D-
(517) Valine, 3-mercapto-, hydrochloride,
       D-
(518) Veratrosine
(519) Veratrum californicum
(520) Veriloid
(521) Vincaleukoblastine   Suspected carcinogen
(522) Vincaleukoblastine, sulfate (1:1)
       (salt)
(523) 3-beta, 20-alpha-Yohimban-16-beta-
       carboxylic acid, 18-beta-hydroxy-11,
       17-alpha-dimethoxy-, methyl ester,
       3, 4, 5-trimethoxybenzoate (ester)   Suspected carcinogen
(524) 3-beta, 20-alpha-Yohimban-16-beta-
       carboxylic acid, 18-beta-hydroxy-
       17-alpha-methoxy-, methyl ester, 3,
       4, 5-trimethoxybenzoate (ester)
(525) Zinc chloride   Suspected carcinogen
(526) Zinc, (ethylenebis(dithiocarbamato))-   Suspected carcinogen
(527) Zinc, (N, N'-propylene-1, 2-bis
       (dithiocarbamate))

APPENDIX II

New Teratogens Reported in 1979 (4) (Not Included in the Appendix I)

(1) Acetaldehyde
(2) Acetamide, 2,2-dichloro-N-(β-hydroxy-α-(hydroxymethyl)-p-nitrophenethyl)-
(3) Acetamide, 2,2-dichloro-N-(β-hydroxy-α-(hydroxymethyl)-p-nitrophenethyl), α ester with sodium succinate
(4) Acetamide, N,N'-octamethylenebis (2,2-dichloro)-
(5) Acetohydroxamic acid, 2-(p-butoxyphenyl)-
(6) 1-Adamantanamine hydrochloride
(7) Ammonium, hexamethylenebis(trimethyl)-, dibromide
(8) Androst-5-ene-3,17-diol,17-methyl-, (3-β,17-β-)
(9) Barbituric acid, 5-ethyl-5-(1-methylbutyl)-2-thio-, sodium salt
(10) Benzenesulfonamide, 4-amino-N-(4,6-dimethoxy-2-pyrimidinyl)-
(11) 3H-1,4-Benzodiazepine, 7-chloro-2-(methylamino)-5-phenyl-,4-oxide
(12) Biphenyl, 2,2'-dichloro-
(13) (1,1'-Biphenyl)-2,2'-diol, 5,5'-dichloro-3,3'-dinitro-
(14) 1,3-Butadiene, hexachloro-
(15) Carbon disulfide
(16) Cholecalciferol, 1a,25-dihydroxy-
(17) Chromium (III) oxide (2:3)
(18) Conium maculatum
(19) 5H-Dibenz(b,f)azepine, 10,11-dihydro-5-(3-(methylamino)propyl)-
(20) 5H-Dibenz(b,f)azepin-2-ol, 10,11-dihydro-5-(3-(dimethylamino)propyl)-
(21) Dibenzo-p-dioxin, 2,7-dichloro-
(22) Dipyrido (1,2-a;2',1'-c)pyrazinediium, 6,7-dihydro-, dibromide
(23) Epipodophyllotoxin, 4'-demethyl-, 9-(4,6-O-2-thenylidene-β-D-glucopyranoside)-

(24) Epipodophyllotoxin-β-D-ethylidenglucoside, 4'demethyl-
(25) Ergotaman-3',6',18-trione, 12'-hydroxy-2',5'-bis(1-methyl-ethyl)-,(5'-α)-, methanesulfonate (salt)
(26) Ethane, 1,1,1-trichloro-2,2-bis(p-methoxyphenyl)-
(27) Ethylene oxide
(28) Formamide, N,N-dimethyl-
(29) Formic acid, methylhydrazide
(30) Glycine, N-formyl-N-hydroxy-, sodium salt
(31) Guanidine, 1-methyl-3-nitro-1-nitroso-
(32) Hydantoin, 5,5-diphenyl,-mixed with 5-ethyl-5-phenylbar-bituric acid (6:1)
(33) Jervine, 3-acetate-
(34) Jervine, N-butyl-12β,13α-dihydro-, 3-acetate-
(35) Jervine, 11-deoxo-12β,13α-dihydro-11α-hydroxy-
(36) Jervine, 12β,13α-dihydro-
(37) Jervine, N-formyl-
(38) Jervine, N-methyl-
(39) Lead
(40) Malonic acid, diethyl ester
(41) Methane, chlorofluoro-
(42) Methanesulfonic acid, ethenyl ester-
(43) Morphinan-3,6-α-diol, 7,8-didehydro-4,5-α-epoxy-17-methyl-, sulfate
(44) Morphinan-6α-ol, 7,8-didehydro-4,5-α-epoxy-3-methoxy-17-methyl-, sulfate (2:1) (salt)
(45) Muldamine
(46) Muldamine, deacetyl-
(47) 2-Naphthacenecarboxamide, 7-chloro-4-(dimethylamino)-1, 4,4a,5,5a,6,11,12a-octahydro-3,6,10,12,12a-pentahydroxy-1, 11-dioxo-
(48) 2-Naphthacenecarboxamide, 4-(dimethylamino)-1,4,4a,5,5a, 6,11,12a-octahydro-3,6,10,12,12a-pentahydroxy-6-methyl-1, 11-dioxo-
(49) Nickel carbonyl
(50) 20-Norcrotalanan-11,15-dione,14,19-dihydro-13-hydroxy-, (12-xi,13-xi)-
(51) 19-Nor-17αpregn-4-en-20-yn-3-one, 17-acetoxy-
(52) 19-Nor-17α-pregnen-20-ynone, 17β-heptanoyloxy-

(53) 19-Nor-17α-pregn-4-en-20-yn-3-one, 17-hydroxy-
(54) 1,2,4-Oxadiazole, 5-(2-(diethylamino)ethyl)-3-phenyl-, citrate
(55) Papain
(56) Phenothiazine, 10-diethylaminopropionyl-3-trifluoromethyl-, hydrochloride
(57) o-Phenylenediamine, 4-nitro-
(58) p-Phenylenediamine, 2-nitro-
(59) Phosphorodithioic acid, O,O-dimethyl ester, S-ester with 2-mercapto-N-methylacetamide
(60) Phosphorothioic acid, O-(2-(ethylthio)ethyl)O,O-dimethyl ester
(61) Picolinic acid, 5-amino-6-(7-amino-6-methoxy-5,8-dioxo-2-quinolyl)-4-(2-hydroxy-3,4-dimethoxyphenyl)-3-methyl-, methyl ester
(62) Picolinic acid, 5-amino-4-(2,3-dihydro-3,4-dimethoxy-2-hydroxyphenyl)-6-(2,2-dimethyl-4-methoxy-5-oxo-5H-imidazo(4,5-h)quinolin-8-yl)-3-methyl-
(63) Piperazine, 1-(p-chloro-α-phenylbenzyl-
(64) Piperazine, 1-(p-chloro-α-phenylbenzyl-, hydrochloride
(65) Piperazine, 1-(p-chloro-α-phenylbenzyl)-4-(m-methylbenzyl)-, hydrochloride
(66) Piperazine, 1-(diphenylmethyl)-4-methyl-, hydrochloride
(67) Polychlorinated biphenyl
(68) Pregna-1,4-diene-2,20-dione,9-fluoro-11β,16α,17,21-tetrahydroxy-,16,21-diacetate
(69) 1,3-Propanediol, 2-amino-2-(hydroxymethyl)-
(70) 2-Propanone, tetrachloro-
(71) 2,4,5,6(1H,3H)-Pyrimidinetetrone, monohydrate
(72) Salicylamide
(73) 5α-Solanidan-3β-ol, (22S,25R)-
(74) Solanid-5-en-3β-ol, (22S,25R)-
(75) Stannane, hydroxytriphenyl-
(76) Streptomycin B
(77) Streptomycin, sulfate (1:3) salt
(78) Thiadiazole
(79) p-Toluamide, N-isopropyl-α-(2-methylhydrazino)-, monohydrochloride
(80) 1-Triazene
(81) s-Triazin-2(1H)-one, 4-amino-1β-D-ribofuranosyl-

(82) 1,2,4-Triazole-3-carboxamide, 1β-D-ribofuranosyl-
(83) Trichothec-9-ene-3α,4β,8α,15-tetrol,12,13-epoxy-, 4,15-diacet-
       ate 8-isovalerate
(84) Triethylamine, 2-(p-(2-chloro-1,2-diphenylvinyl)phenoxy)-,
       citrate, (E)-
(85) Uracil, 6-propyl-2-thio-
(86) Zinc sulfate (1:1)

REFERENCES

1. Shepard, T. H.: *Catalog of Teratogenic Agents.* Baltimore, Maryland, The Johns Hopkins Univ. Press, 1973, pp. xi-xiv.
2. Kolb Meyers, V., and Meyers, C. Y.: *Chemicals Which Cause Birth Defects-Teratogens. A Brief Guide.* Carbondale, Illinois, Southern Illinois University, 1980; available from the authors at cost ($3.00).
3. *Registry of Toxic Effects of Chemical Substances,* by National Institute for Occupational Safety and Health. Available as printed edition (updated annually), microfiche issue (updated quarterly), and on-line computer data base (updated quarterly).
4. *"Tumorigenic, Teratogenic, and Mutagenic Citations: Subfiles of the Registry of Toxic Effects of Chemical Substances",* by National Institute for Occupational Safety and Health, 1979 (microfiche).
5. Shepard, T. H., Miller, J. R., and Marois, M. (Eds.): *Methods for Detection of Environmental Agents that Produce Congenital Defects.* New York, New York, American Elsevier Publ., Co., Inc., 1975. pp. 29–48 (Ch. 5, by Wilson, J. G.).
6. *ibid,* pp. 79–88 (Ch. 7 by Zimmerman, E. F.).
7. *ibid,* pp. 65–77 (Ch. 6, by Schumacher, H. J.).
8. *CRC Handbook of Chemistry and Physics,* 60th Edition, Boca Raton, Florida, CRC Press, Inc., 1979, pp. C–1 to C–58.
9. IUPAC tentative rules for the nomenclature of organic chemistry. Section E. Fundamental stereochemistry. *J Org Chem, 35:*2849–2867, 1970.
10. IUPAC-IUB revised tentative rules for nomenclature of steroids. *Biochemistry, 8:*2227–2242, 1969.
11. *The Merck Index,* Ninth Edition, Merck and Co., Inc., Rahway, New Jersey, 1976.
12. Nishimura, H., and Tanimura, T.: *Clinical Aspects of the Teratogenicity of Drugs.* New York, American Elsevier Publ., Co., Inc., 1976, pp. 99–259.
13. Wijnne, H.: in Buisman, J. A. K. (Ed.): *Biological Activity and Chemical Structure.* New York, New York, Elsevier Publ., 1977, pp. 211–229.
14. Schulster, D., and Levitzki, A., (Eds.): *Cellular Receptors.* New York, New York, John Wiley and Sons, 1980, pp. 91–125 (Ch. 6 by Mainwaring, W. I. P.).
15. *ibid,* pp. 309–330 (Ch. 17 by Miller, R. J.).
16. Korolkovas, A.: *Essentials of Molecular Pharmacology.* New York, New York, Wiley-Interscience Publ., 1970, pp. 8–10.
17. Walters, D. B. (Ed.): *Safe Handling of Chemical Carcinogens, Mutagens, Teratogens and Highly Toxic Substances,* Vol. 1 and 2. Ann Arbor, Michigan, Ann Arbor Science Publishers, Inc., 1980.

Chapter 9

ENVIRONMENTAL REGULATORY PROGRAM FOR TOXIC POLLUTANTS TODAY AND TOMORROW

Mike Mauzy

What is meant by a toxic pollutant? The United States Environmental Protection Agency criteria for classification as a toxic pollutant include the following:

1. Evidence of acute or chronic effects on humans or terrestrial life;
2. Persistence including morbidity and environmental degradability;
3. Bioaccumulation factors;
4. Synergistic propensies and effects; and
5. Effects, persistence, and bioaccumulation of degradation products and metabolites of the parent compound.

Toxic effects may be classified as acute or chronic, and both measurements are significant factors in safely regulating human exposure to toxics. Also the effects of the materials are characterized by the extent of the injury. Frequently these classifications of effects are as follows:

1. Reversible,
2. Nonreversible, and
3. Irreversible.

Because of the breadth of scope of this subject, some constraints are placed on the balance of the following remarks. For this purpose, toxic pollutants do not include any radioactive material, high level radioactive waste, spent nuclear fuel or low level radiological waste. These materials are excluded from this subject because the solution to the issues and concerns from these materials are very different from the solution to these issues and concerns of chemical toxicants. The chronic effects are the primary concern because they can be and frequently are, delayed for years after exposure. The acute effects of toxic materials and pollutants are today seldom experienced other than in accidental releases, incidents, or emergency situations. When they do occur, they normally involve, impact, and expose a limited population and do not result in exposure to the general public.

In this context, toxic pollutants are a concern, a sensative subject, or a cause for fear depending upon one's level of knowledge and the perspectives that result from his role and responsibility in relation to toxic pollutants and toxic materials. No one is neutral on the issue of exposure to toxic pollutants; exposure comes from products consumed or used, work places, and the environment. In everyday life, we are exposed, sometimes knowingly, frequently unknowingly. For these reasons few people today question the desirability of and need for controls on the exposure to toxic materials and toxic pollutants.

Public *awareness* of the presence and the effects of exposure to toxic materials and toxic pollutants has grown significantly in the past five years. No one working in a public capacity who is exposed to the media can doubt the interest and concern in this pervasive issue. KEPONE, PCB, PBB, and DIOXIN are now household words that create negative images, almost always with consequences approaching that of a disaster. Love Canal, Valley of the Drums, and the other such incidents are perceived by the public to be the normal situation rather than isolated examples, and it is just a matter of time before many other equally serious situations are discovered.

Public *concern* about toxic chemicals in the environment and the disposal of industrial hazardous waste in 1980 is very substantial. In a recent national public opinion poll, 64 percent expressed a great deal of concern about the disposal of industrial hazardous chemical wastes. *This is a higher level of concern than has been expressed for air or water pollution in any public opinion survey since 1970.* This same opinion survey reported that 83 percent of the respondents felt that all chemicals should be screened prior to their commercial use and believed that the government should conduct an extensive screening program to make sure that all chemicals are safe before they are used. It is now common knowledge that we are living in an era of antiregulatory sentiment. It is also important to understand that this sentiment does not apply regulatory programs to control exposure to toxic materials and toxic pollutants. The public is concerned and fearful of the effects of exposure to these materials on the health of the current population and the effects of such exposure on future generations.

In this emotionally charged atmosphere, it is not necessary to justify the merits and benefits of a regulatory program. Public support for such programs exists and the public is demanding a rapid governmental response. The main task then is to develop and implement a program that is effective both in its delivery system and in the results it produces. Further challenge is to develop and implement a program that is credible to the public and to our professional responsibilities. This is the only path to continuing public support for programs to regulate or control toxic materials and toxic pollutants in the environment.

Today, we have regulatory programs conducted by the Occupational Safety and Health Administration to control exposure in the work place. There are also programs carried out by the United States Environmental Protection Agency and state pollution control agencies to control toxic pollutants in the environment. However there are no programs at present for the control of exposure in homes, and this is an emerging issue that will be addressed in the years to come.

The United States Environmental Protection Agency has a virtual arsenal of regulatory control programs to deal with toxic pollutants in the environment. There are programs on air pollution, water pollution, public water supply, waste disposal, and the control of manufacturing, distributing and use of toxic materials.

Section 112 of the Clean Air Act established a program of national emission standards for hazardous air pollutants. This program establishes technology based emission standards for hazardous air pollutants. These emission standards apply to both new facilities that are constructed as well as to existing facilities that emit any of the listed pollutants. At the present time, the United

States Environmental Protection Agency has listed asbestos, beryllium, mercury, and vinylchloride under this section of the Clean Air Act, and emissions of these materials are now regulated. This approach requires listing of each material compound by compound and is a very arduous standard setting process that will prove ineffective for any widespread control program for toxic air pollutants.

The Toxic Substances Control Act seeks to exercise control over chemical substances and mixtures whose manufacture, processing, and distribution in commerce, use, or disposal may present an unreasonable risk of injury to health or the environment. This act applies to all new products that are produced as well as to existing products in commerce and use. The act seeks to require the development of adequate data on the effects of the chemical substances, including mixtures, on health and the environment. Following an evaluation of the data, the Administrator of the United States Environmental Protection Agency is empowered to bring the material under regulatory control to restrict or prohibit its use or distribution.

The authority of the Toxic Substances Control Act is a powerful tool and the Environmental Protection Agency is currently in the early stages of developing and implementing programs to exercise the authorities granted by Congress. *An effective future toxic pollutant control program will be strictly a reactive one unless the Toxic Substances Control Act is effectively and aggressively implemented.* All of the other control programs are reactive because they seek to control a toxic pollutant as it enters the environment or after it has already entered the environment.

The Safe Drinking Water Act seeks to regulate the quality of potable water for human consumption throughout the nation. This act further seeks to protect ground water sources from contamination where those ground water sources are currently used as raw water sources for water supplies or where they may be used as such in the future. Certainly potable water is one product that is consumed and is a potential source of exposure to toxic pollutants. At the present time, public water supplies are being analyzed for a wide range of organic and inorganic toxicants and, where excessive concentrations are found, steps are taken to provide necessary treatment to the water prior to its delivery into the distribution system. This program is an important monitoring program, but will not be effective in controlling exposure to toxic pollutants.

The Resource Conservation and Recovery Act provides a regulatory control program for the disposal of hazardous wastes that result primarily from the technological society. This program can be very effective in assuring destruction, immobilization, and long-term disposal of the industrial by-products so that they will not present future threats to the environment or to public health. The program began with the initial phases becoming effective November 19, 1980.

The Clean Water Act provides authority for the control of toxic pollutants discharged into sewer systems or discharged from treatment plants into the streams and rivers on the nation. This program was created by the National Resources Defense Council consent decree and was codified in the Clean Water Act by the Congress in 1977. The program is just now becoming operational and it is too early to tell whether it will be effective.

Because it is an older more mature program, the National Water Quality Program and the discharge and pretreatment programs for toxic pollutants are carried out under the Clean Water Act. The basic thrust is the promulgation of a priority pollutant list and a list of primary industries to be controlled. The industries for control are selected on the basis of their probability of producing in their waste streams one or more of the priority pollutants. Also, the United States Environmental Protection Agency is in the process of developing instream water quality standards for the priority pollutants using associated criteria of (1) "no effect" levels for aquatic life with no consideration of varying species tolerance and (2) human health protection associated with substantial consumption of both the water and the indigenous fish and shell fish.

The Illinois Environmental Protection Agency has several major concerns about the data and theory associated with the criteria used in adopting the federal standards. However, some of the problems relate to establishing standards to protect drinking water when no potential public water supply exists. These are only a few of the shortcomings of the broad reaching resource intensive priority pollutant approach. The resulting monitoring programs required both of the regulatory agency and the dischargers are significant and are applicable even when no real potential for the presence of any given pollutant exists. There is no need to make broad generalizations based on industrial categories and speculations on the impacts of pretreatment.

The federal pretreatment regulations are also all encompassing and impractical. To date, the regulations have proven to be confusing if not overwhelming for both the state and the substate treatment plant owners. The problem assessment, present technology, and time limitations do not warrent the far-reaching toxics program envisioned by the federal pretreatment regulations.

A survey performed by the Illinois Environmental Protection Agency in the spring of 1979 revealed that of the major publicly owned facilities that process over five million gallons per day, 93 percent had existing ordinances to regulate industrial flows into their sewer systems, 32 percent had some problems with industrial discharges into their systems, and 25 percent had discharge violations attributable to industrial waste.

It is important to note that an estimated 78 percent of all of the indirect industrial dischargers in the state are tributary to these major facilities. The only thing wrong with the present programs is that they have not been given an opportunity to work. Thus, the local governments must be more diligent in enforcing existing ordinances. The federal pretreatment program nonetheless requires that these past actions be set aside and entirely new programs be put into place.

Illinois has pursued the fundamental precept that its regulatory control programs must be founded upon sound technical principles and analysis. This has proven to be a very demanding, but rewarding canon. It is from this rigorous technical perspective that the Illinois Environmental Protection Agency incrementally approached the problem of controlling toxic substances. What the agency has learned has been most useful and productive, and what it does not know draws it forward to greater levels of technical sophistication and program refinement. Where the agency is comfortable with the state of knowledge, it aggressively implements the control programs, and where it is faced with too many questions and unknowns, open-minded scientific studies are initiated. The agency believes the results achieved to date support the soundness of this strategy.

It should also be mentioned at the outset that a correlary assumption associated with the toxic strategy is the approach taken by the agency essentially precludes the notion that formal regulatory programs are an appropriate mechanism for forcing or driving technological innovation. The Agency contends that pollutant reduction is principally a function of the treatability of the compound or property to be controlled rather than the industrial category from which the pollutant originates. Therefore, the standards and control strategies apply equally to all. The Agency does not preclude the benefits of improved practices and manufacturing processes.

The development of a scientific, valid toxic substances program and strategy requires program elements be in place and functioning. These include the following:

1. Expertise in quality control and quality assurance,
2. Statistical expertise,
3. Indepth understanding of the requirements imposed by different sampling procedures,
4. Mathematical tools for relating and integrating biological and chemical data, and
5. A good understanding of environmental quality and environmental interactions.

As an indication of the commitment to action, the agency laboratories alone conduct about 50,000 organic chemical analyses per year. This number is projected to increase to over 250,000 analyses per year by 1985. Add to this analytical capability approximately 500,000 analyses performed yearly on inorganic parameters such as heavy metals, cyanide and the more conventional environmental parameters.

The commitment to extensive monitoring and analysis of all forms of pollution is clear. The laboratory staff is continuously in touch with the United States Environmental Protection Agency research labs to assure that the analytical methods and equipment are providing the most accurate and sensitive results possible. In addition to the inhouse program, the agency participates in quality assurance programs carried out by the United States Environmental Protection Agency, the United States General Services, and the United States Food and Drug Administration.

In the near future, toxic pollutant control programs will be carried out using existing regulatory tools available to the United States Environmental Protection Agency and to the states. In pursuing this course of action, Illinois will be constantly making resource trade-offs because the present direction of the program requires such significant resource inputs in terms of trained manpower, funding and time that the programs cannot and will not be effectively implemented. In many cases, sampling methodologies and protocols must be developed, as well improved, more sensitive analytical methods. Once the agency is able to more effectively monitor for the presence of toxic pollutants in the environment, other data needs will become necessary.

More data and information is necessary in assessing the risk of exposure to toxics. Risk of exposure is a factor, but acceptability of risk is another equally important factor, a factor that depends upon benefits derived, the nature of the population exposed, and the availability of practical alternatives. It is not possible to guarantee a risk-free society, however we must recognize that risks imposed on persons who gain no benefit are generally not acceptable. Personal choice and personal values enter into a risk/benefit comparison, and each person must be allowed the widest possible choice supported by full information on risks as well as benefits so that intelligent choices can be made.

The use and application of safety factors in establishing limits on our control programs must be subject to increasing scrutiny. Classical toxicology shows that, for many toxic substances, the frequency of a toxic effect declines as the dosage declines. We must understand the response relationships more fully, and we must ascertain whether a threshold for toxic pollutants exists, such that there is a positive, unobservable effect level. At the present time, scientific information is not completely available to respond to these issues. Therefore, in the meantime implementation of toxic controls strategy is based on conservative, perhaps illfounded assumptions.

As the current program directions are implemented, specific steps should be taken to insure that the data gaps are filled. Hopefully in the near future, the priority pollutant laundry list and the compound by compound regulatory strategy will be reconsidered. Research must be initiated to promote and build valid, technical and scientific foundations for the program prior to implementation of full-scale regulatory control programs. In the meantime, we should be pursuing nonregulatory approaches to promoting the advancement of technology relating to toxic materials and toxic pollutants. Increased effort must be devoted to the development of reliable data base information from which valid technical assessments can be made. The type, quality, and quantity of data needed to answer specific questions must be identified. The appropriate data must be collected, analyzed, and properly interpreted.

In summary, toxic pollutants in the environment today are a problem and are a concern of significance to the public. The public demands a response, and, accordingly, government is responding by developing and implementing regulatory control programs to reduce exposure to toxic pollutants. It is believed that the control programs being developed today are based on inadequate technical information, poorly conceived, and unimplementable. It is an earnest hope that sufficient scientific studies will be initiated and that they can be completed in time to make midcourse corrections from the current program directions in order to refine and redirect the programs.

Chapter 10

EPA POLICIES TO PROTECT THE HEALTH OF CONSUMERS OF DRINKING WATER IN THE UNITED STATES

Joseph A. Cotruvo

ABSTRACT

In the United States, the objective is to protect drinking water at the source, during treatment, and during distribution. In 1975, interim regulations for bacteria and turbidity, ten inorganic chemicals, six organic chemicals, and radionuclides were promulgated. In 1979, National Secondary Regulations for substances affecting the aesthetic quality of water were promulgated. In 1979, trihalomethanes were added. The United States Environmental Protection Agency (U.S. EPA) is engaged in comprehensive revisions of the National Primary Drinking Water Regulations.

The areas of the most significant concern include detection and control of contamination of ground waters by organic chemicals resulting from improper disposal practices, a reassessment of microbiological regulations and toxicity of disinfectant by-products, and a major effort to deal with corrosion-related contamination of drinking water during distribution. The evaluation of the issue of a granular activated carbon requirement for contaminated surface waters is under consideration. A program to assure the quality of direct and indirect additives to drinking water has also been

This paper was presented to the International Workshop on Water Supply and Health, Amsterdam, 1980. Prepared on government time, this chapter may be reprinted royalty free for U.S. Government purposes.

initiated. Part of this activity will include determination of the contaminants and by-products associated with the use of various water treatment chemicals and pipe materials.

INTRODUCTION

The objective is to assure that drinking water is a safe and high quality commodity that is, to the extent feasible, free from agents that can cause harm to the public. Our drinking waters do, in general, meet that objective, however, there are concerns that demand continued vigilance to protect drinking water, and study to determine the extent that the existence of trace contaminants may contribute to public health risks.

This paper deals with a number of the activities and policies of the U.S. EPA's Office of Drinking Water in carrying out the mandates of the Safe Drinking Water Act of 1974 including past, current and future regulatory actions, guidelines, emergency response actions, and a new program to assure the quality of additives to drinking water during treatment and distribution.

The Drinking Water Cycle

It is well known that substantial contamination of drinking water can occur at any point in the cycle that includes the raw water source, the treatment process and during distribution.

SOURCE PROTECTION: A number of mechanisms are available to control the introduction of contaminants into raw water. These include legislation to control industrial waste discharges and hazardous waste disposal, and controls on the introduction into commerce and uses of chemicals. The major pieces of legislation in the United States for these purposes include the 1972 Federal Water Pollution Control Act (Clean Water Act) and later amendments, the Resource Conservation and Recovery Act of 1976, the Toxic Substances Control Act, and the Federal Insecticide, Fungicide and Rodenticide Act.

WATER TREATMENT: As water treatment is applied for the essential purpose of purifying contaminated waters, the addition of treatment chemicals can in fact add contaminants, and the by-products of the reactions of some treatment chemicals in water are also contaminants. The more raw water is contaminated, the more extensive the treatment needed to purify it and the greater the demand for chemical additives. Regulations for trihalomethanes (THMs) have been issued (i.e. 0.10 mg/l total trihalomethanes). Maximum Contaminant Levels (MCLs) in finished water for inorganic and organic chemicals also indirectly constrain the quality, quantity, and type of source treatment chemicals. A new direct and indirect additives quality evaluation and control program is being established.

DISTRIBUTION SYSTEMS: Corrosion of pipe surfaces is the major source of lead and cadmium and some other metals in finished drinking water. Additional MCLs and a corrosion control program are being initiated under the Safe Drinking Water Act and the indirect additives program will also be effective here.

The Safe Drinking Water Act

In 1974, the Safe Drinking Water Act[1] was passed so that the public throughout the country could be assured of receiving drinking water that at least met minimum uniform quality criteria. The law applies to all public water systems, which are defined as those that serve drinking water regularly to 25 persons or consist of at least fifteen service connections. Community water systems are those public water systems that serve resident populations at least 60 days out of the year. There are at least 60,000 community water systems and perhaps 300,000 noncommunity systems in the United States. Approximately 200 million people are served by these community systems. The vast majority of systems are small (between 25 to 500 persons) (Figure 10–1), however, they include only 2 percent of the population. The approximately 2700 large systems (greater than 10,000), although only 5 percent of the systems, serve about 80 percent of the population. The law applies equally to small and large systems, however, very different problems need to be faced in each type of system. As expected, small systems are limited in their capability to control drinking water quality by their small financial base, and lack of access to technical services and qualified operating personnel.

The Safe Drinking Water Act is a complex law, but basically it consists of the following tenets:

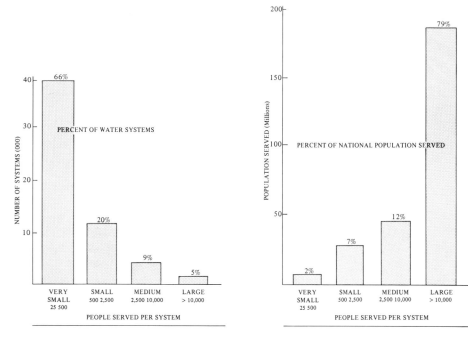

Figure 10–1. The majority of community water systems are very small . . . The larger systems serve the vast majority of the population.

1. EPA must identify substances in drinking water that *may* have an adverse effect on health.
2. EPA must then establish MCLs to protect health that will control those chemicals to the extent feasible, taking costs and other factors into consideration. However, if monitoring for a substance is not technically and economically feasible, treatment technology should be specified that will reduce levels to the extent feasible.

According to the law, the sequence of events to be followed for implementation are as follows:

1. National Interim Primary Drinking Water Standards and National Secondary Standards
2. National Academy of Sciences Report with *recommended* MCLs
3. List of Contaminants and Goal Levels that would result in "no known or anticipated adverse effect on health"

4. MCLs or Treatment Requirements (Revised National Primary Drinking Water (Regulations)

National Interim Primary Drinking Water Regulations

Comprehensive National Interim Primary Drinking Water Regulations (NIPDWR) were published in December, 1975, and became effective in June, 1977.[2] They consisted of MCLs for ten inorganic substances, six organic pesticides, radionuclides, coliform bacteria, and turbidity. These regulations include monitoring requirements and analytical methods (Table 10–I).

These interim regulations were amended, in 1979, to include an MCL for total trihalomethanes.[3] In August, 1980, they were amended again to include a requirement to monitor for sodium (not an MCL) and initiation of actions to deal with corrosive waters by

Table 10–I

NATIONAL INTERIM PRIMARY DRINKING WATER REGULATIONS

Arsenic	0.05 mg/l
Barium	1.0 mg/l
Cadmium	0.010 mg/l
Chromium	0.05 mg/l
Lead	0.05 mg/l
Mercury	0.002 mg/l
Nitrate (as N)	10 mg/l
Selenium	0.01 mg/l
Silver	0.05 mg/l
Fluoride	1.4–2.4 mg/l (ambient temp)
Endrin	0.002 mg/l
Lindane	0.004 mg/l
Methoxychlor	0.1 mg/l
Toxaphene	0.005 mg/l
2, 4-D	0.1 mg/l
2, 4, 5-TP Silvex	0.01 mg/l
Coliform bacteria	< 1 per 100 ml
Radium–226 + radium − 228	5 pCi/l
Gross alpha particle activity	15 pCi/l
Beta particle and photon radioactivity	4 mrem (annual dose equivalent)
Turbidity	1 Tu (up to 5 Tu)
Trihalomethanes (the sum of concentrations of bromodichloromethane, dibromochloromethane, tribromomethane (bromoform) and trichloromethane (chloroform)	0.10 mg/l

Table 10-II

NATIONAL SECONDARY DRINKING WATER REGULATIONS

Chloride	250 mg/l
Color	15 color units
Copper	1 mg/l
Corrosivity	Non-corrosive
Foaming Agents	0.5 mg/l
Iron	0.3 mg/l
Manganese	0.05 mg/l
Odor	3 threshold odor number
pH	6.5–8.5
Sulfate	250 mg/l
TDS	500 mg/l
Zinc	5 mg/l

requiring identification of pipe materials and analyses for corrosion related factors such as pH, alkalinity, and hardness.

National Secondary Regulations were also published in 1979.[4] These are actually guidance for the states rather than regulations since they are not federally enforceable, as opposed to primary regulations. Secondary regulations deal with factors that affect the aesthetic qualities of drinking water: taste, odor, color (Table 10–II).

The Safe Drinking Water Act (SDWA) includes a timetable leading to Revised National Primary Drinking Water Regulations. The National Academy of Sciences (NAS) is to provide a series of reports to advise EPA in development of the revised regulations. According to the SDWA, the NAS is to produce a number of "Recommended MCLs" from which EPA is to develop a list of health goal levels of contaminants that would result in "no known or anticipated adverse effects on health." Revised regulations would be derived from these recommended MCLs by incorporating technological and economic feasibility factors. Treatment requirements would also be derived for those substances for which monitoring is not technologically and economically feasible.

"Drinking Water and Health," the first NAS report, did not contain those recommended MCLs, thus, EPA's work has been dedicated to develop the information needed to produce revised primary regulations. These are expected to be proposed within two years.

The NAS report did provide a number of principles that EPA has adopted as matters of policy to be applied in the development of information on health risks from contaminants in drinking water (Table 10–III).[5]

These principles do not, of course, in themselves determine standards, because standards include factors of technological and economic feasibility. They do, however, provide a basis for interpretation of the health effects data and in assessing the human risks.

Regulation Development Process

Table 10–IV is an illustration of the administration and procedural aspects of our process for developing regulations and the types of background documentation that must be developed before a drinking water regulation can be completed.

Typically, the entire process may require three to five years from initiation to completion.

Organic Chemicals

Organic chemicals are just one group of contaminants that are found in drinking water that have received substantial investigation. There are four categories of organic chemical contamination with which EPA is dealing: surface water, ground water, disinfection process and additives (see Table 10–V).

Going beyond pollution control activities, a number of control approaches are being developed under SDWA authorities.

Surface water contaminants will be dealt with through MCLs for individual chemicals and through treatment improvements that will effectively remove broad groups of contaminants (e.g. improved coagulation, filtration and activated carbon).

Ground water contaminants are being detected with greater frequency and often at levels that far exceed those found in surface waters. Improper waste disposal practices of the past are now

Table 10–III

NAS PRINCIPLES

1. Effects in animals properly qualified are applicable to man.

2. Methods do not now exist to establish a threshold for long-term effects of toxic agents.

3. Exposure of experimental animals to toxic agents in high doses is a necessary and valid method of discovering possible carcinogenic hazards in man.

4. Material should be assessed in terms of human risk, rather than as "safe" or "unsafe."

Table 10–IV

REGULATION DEVELOPMENT

Technical Assessments
  Exposure Assessment
    Occurrence of Contaminants in Drinking Water
    Routes of Exposure (Body Burden)
  Health Criteria
  Analytical Methods
  Monitoring Requirements and Costs
  Treatment Technology and Costs
  Economic Impact Assessment
  Regional and State Resource Analysis
Preparation of Rule-making Package
  Option/Decision Memoranda
  Preamble/Regulation
  Action Memo to Administrator
  Statement of Basis and Purpose
  Treatment Manual
  Economic Impact Document
Review Process
  Outside Reviews (e.g. Regions, States, American Water Works Association, Environmental
    Defense Fund)
  EPA Work Group
  Assistant Administrator Approval
  Steering Committee
  Red Border Review
  Federal Register Notice
  Comment Period Public Hearing
  Review Comments
  Prepare Rule-making Package
  Begin Review Process

leading to drinking water source contamination often at levels that far exceed those found in surface waters; levels that necessitate abandonment of wells or installation of extensive treatment. The most commonly found contaminants to date appear to be chlorinated methane and ethane (ethylene) derivatives, which share the properties of being very high volume industrial chemicals (millions of kilograms per year), very widespread use, high biological and chemical stability, and hydrophobicity; thus, they bind poorly to sediments and migrate in the ground more rapidly than many other chemicals.

EPA is currently developing MCLs for a number of these substances and expects an Advance Notice of Proposed Rulemaking

Table 10–V

ORGANIC CHEMICALS IN DRINKING WATER

Surface Water	Natural Products
	Industrial Effluents
	Municipal Effluents
	Urban and Rural Runoff
Ground Water	Natural Products
	Industrial Waste and Landfills
	Septic Tanks
	Pesticides
Disinfection	Disinfection By-products
Additives	Treatment Chemicals
	Paints and Coatings
	Pipes

(ANPRM) to be published before the end of 1981 for most of the following list: trichloroethylene, tetrachlorethylene, 1,2-dichloroethane, 1,1,1-trichloroethane, carbon tetrachloride, vinyl chloride, dichloroethylene, methylene chloride and 1,1-dichloroethane. Extensive treatment technology development work is underway. It now appears that granular activated carbon, aeration and possibly macroreticular resins are the technologies that will find the greatest application in those small water systems that are most often affected by ground water contamination.

DISINFECTION — By-products of the oxidation processes used for disinfection have been shown to introduce relatively large amounts of organic chemicals primarily by reaction of the oxidant (e.g. chlorine, ozone, or chlorine dioxide) with organic chemicals. In the United States, work has tended to concentrate on the by-products of chlorination, since chlorine is the most heavily applied disinfectant. The trihalomethanes (chloroform, bromoform, bromodichloromethane, dibromochloromethane) are the by-products that have been regulated by an MCL of 0.10 mg/l.

Disinfection is acknowledged to be one of the most significant public health protection processes ever developed, thus control of disinfection by-products must never be construed in any way to reduce disinfection practice or efficiency. Rather improper practices, such as applying uncontrolled amounts of chlorine to insufficiently pretreated waters have been shown to unnecessarily add large amounts of by-product chemicals to finished drinking water.

THM levels in some drinking waters in the United States have been found approaching 1000 μg/l, yet THMs are only a portion of the by-products that are produced; a recent survey by EPA's Office of Drinking Water of fifty drinking waters found that THMs ranged from 10 percent to 90 percent of total organic halogen concentrations.[6] In addition, the organochlorine compounds are only a portion of the total oxidation by-products of disinfection. Therefore, U.S. EPA considers THMs to be an easily measured indicator of the presence of a host of additional by-products as well as chemicals that should be controlled on their own merit.

In summary, THMs are regulated because—

1. drinking water is the major source of human exposure to these chemicals and their associated by-products;
2. they are the most ubiquitous synthetic organic chemicals found in drinking water in the United States;
3. they are normally found in the largest quantity among synthetics (surface waters);
4. they are produced during water treatment and thus they are controllable by normal technologies;
5. health risks are indicated by high dose animal tests; and
6. they are indicative of many other by-products concurrently found.

Any disinfectant is a drinking water additive and can produce a variety of by-products. EPA is stressing research studies to determine the possible risks associated with exposure to all common disinfectants and their by-products.

ADDITIVES—Direct and indirect additives (Table 10–VI) are another voluntary source of chemicals in drinking water that should be considered contaminants when present in excessive or unnecessary amounts.

EPA is developing an additive control program by creating a Branch unit within the Criteria and Standards Division. The authorities for such a program were established in 1980 and the new program is expected to initiate operation in mid-1982.[7] Program segments now being developed include:

1. Establishment of policies and administrative procedures;

Table 10–VI
CATEGORIES OF ADDITIVES

DIRECT
    Treatment Chemicals
    Insecticides
    Herbicides
    Corrosion Control Chemicals
    Evaporative Suppressants
    Fluorescent Dyes
    Coagulant Aids

INDIRECT
    Detergents
    Sanitizers
    Joint Lubricants
    Asphaltic Liners
    Concrete Coatings
    Plastic and Rubber Liners
    Paint Liners

2. Purity criteria (Water Chemicals Codex);
3. Development of simulated use tests for surfaces;
4. Risk assessment criteria;
5. Create an information system;
6. Lift the current moratorium on new applications; and
7. Begin a systematic review of old approvals.

Emergency Response

In addition to the establishment of long-term policies and programs and regulations, there exists a need to deal with drinking
water problems resulting from contamination by chemicals that
are not regulated, and also from short-term contamination such as
from spills that may cause risks of acute toxicity. The Criteria and
Standards Division has developed an emergency advisory program
that produces documents called SNARLs that contain detailed
information and advice of importance to state and local organiza-
tions who must make a determination of potability. SNARL stands
for *Suggested No Adverse Response Level*, a term coined by the NAS
Safe Drinking Water Committee. The SNARL document usually
consists of several pages of discussion of the toxicology of the

substances, then presents recommended drinking water levels that would result in negligible risk under several exposure conditions along with the complete method of computation.

Acute Toxicity   — 1 day
Subchronic   — 7–10 days
Chronic   — long-term
Carcinogenicity — lifetime risks

Acute, subchronic, and chronic toxicity values are computed by classical toxicological practice beginning with the experimental highest no adverse effects or lowest adverse effect level in animals with an applied safety factor. For a carcinogen, the same computations are made based upon noncarcinogenic toxicology, but, in addition, quantitative incremental lifetime risks are also stated for daily exposures equivalent to one in 100,000 and one in 1 million risks are provided. These are computed by the conservative linear nonthreshold multistage risk model discussed by the NAS in their 1977 report *Drinking Water and Health.*[8]

The program has been very successful and encouraged by many states and local water utilities. Thus far, SNARLs have been developed for eight chemicals including tri- and tetrachloroethylene, kerosene, diesel oil, and several pesticides. Approximately twenty more SNARLs are expected to be developed this year.

Future Actions

EPA's main efforts in drinking water quality assurance in the future will concentrate on the development of comprehensive Revised National Primary Drinking Water Regulations. These will require a complete reevaluation of all existing interim regulations and those expected to be proposed in 1983. Before the end of 1981, MCLs for a number of organohalogen contaminants primarily affecting ground water will be proposed. It is essential that these proceed rapidly because of the widespread contamination by these substances being detected. Major research efforts investigating the toxicology of disinfectant chemicals and their by-products in water are under way, which will likely lead to more comprehensive controls in addition to the existing THM regulations. A new program to evaluate direct and indirect additives to drinking water is in development and expected to be initiated in 1981. Suggested No Adverse Response Level (SNARL) recommendations for a large number of additional contaminants are expected in 1980 and 1981. Particular emphasis will be placed on dealing with the unique problems faced by small public water systems both in obtaining and operating the technology to achieve high quality drinking water, but also addressing their financial limitations.

Thus, a large number of ambitious programs are underway. Each of these fit within the master plan to fully implement the Safe Drinking Water Act and assure the quality of drinking water in the United States.

References

1. Safe Drinking Water Act, as amended, 42 U.S.C. 300f *et seq.*
2. National Interim Primary Drinking Water Regulations, 40 CFR 141.
3. National Interim Primary Drinking Water Regulations; Control of Trihalomethanes in Drinking Water, 44 *FR* 68624.
4. National Secondary Drinking Water Regulations, 40 CFR 143.
5. Drinking Water and Health, A Report of the Safe Drinking Water Committee, National Academy of Sciences, 1977. Chapter II. Chemical Contaminants: Safety and Risk Assessment, pp. 53-58.
6. Personal Communication from Stig Regli and Duncan MacKeever.
7. Drinking Water Technical Assistance; Implementation Plan for Control of Direct and Indirect Additives to Drinking Water and Memorandum of Understanding Between the Environmental Protection Agency and the Food and Drug Administration, 44 *FR* 42775.
8. Drinking Water and Health, A Report of the Safe Drinking Water Committee, National Academy of Sciences, 1977. Chapter II, pp. 47-49.

Chapter 11

BIVALVES AS MONITORS FOR PERSISTENT POLLUTANTS IN MARINE AND FRESHWATER ENVIRONMENTS

JAMES B. JOHNSTON AND DEAN M. HARTLEY

INTRODUCTION

North American surface waters, estuarine, and coastal waters have served as the receptacle of vast quantities of man-produced, petroleum-derived chemicals, especially since the beginning of the "chemical era" in the United States after World War II. Man's activities have released an enormous variety of chemicals to these waters from industrial and municipal effluents, from runoff of treated agricultural lands, landfill leachates and dumps, fallout of compounds formed during incineration of materials, and spills and deliberate dumping of wastes into streams and on the continental shelf. Although a substantial fraction of these chemicals are degraded by physical or biological processes in the aquatic environment, a number of persistent ones remain that are refractory to natural degradative processes. Indeed, some of the most important of these biorefractory or recalcitrant compounds were deliberately manufactured for their environmental persistence. Among these are the persistent pesticides, biocidal compounds intended to kill plants, insects, or animals. The persistence permitted the biocidal effects to be obtained for a full growing season with only one or a few applications.

Originally, the persistence of these compounds was not thought to present any particular hazard, even though the persistent pesticides are clearly toxic. Safety was assumed because (a) pesticides and other materials discharged into the environment are diluted by percolation into the soil, flow into rivers and ultimately flow into the oceans and (b) the primary axiom of toxicology teaches that toxicity is related first of all to concentration: everything is toxic at a high enough dose.[1] Therefore the toxicity of persistent compounds was thought to be mitigated by dilution in the environment.

It happens, however, that the chemical structures that tend to be resistent to biodegradation frequently impart hydrophobic and lipophilic properties to a compound. Lipophilic compounds tend to be retained efficiently by organisms at each step in a food chain. Thus persistent, hydrophobic compounds present in the aquatic environment tend to accumulate and to be concentrated in organisms at the top of food chains that begin with simple aquatic organisms. This is the phenomenon of ecological magnification.[2] Because of ecological magnification, toxic compounds may occur in the top feeders of a food chain in concentrations that may cause overt toxic effects. In the past, persistent compounds were often released into the environment with no regard for their potential ecological magnification and without knowledge of their effects in natural food webs.

BIVALVES AS POLLUTION MONITORS

Recognition of the declining quality of many of the nation's fresh waters—with extreme examples such as Lake Erie—led the United States Congress to pass sweeping environmental protection legislation at the height of the environmental movement in the early 1970s. Typical of this legislation is the Federal Water Pollution Control Act of 1972 (Public Law 92-500 and its amendments) which mandates the restoration and maintenance of the integrity of United States waters. This legislation specifically calls for water quality sufficient to protect wildlife, fish, and shellfish. It presents a challenge to aquatic biologists and chemists; how can they best monitor the quality of the aquatic environment and how can they detect toxic and/or persistent pollutants that might affect aquatic life? In addition, how can the monitoring be accomplished at reasonable expense and convenience while maintaining sensitivity to a broad range of pollutants?

One innovative technique that responds to many of these concerns is the analysis of bivalve molluscs. In 1978, Phillips suggested the following criteria for good biological monitors of water quality[3]: (1) the organism should bioaccumulate pollutants above environmental levels, but should not be killed at these levels, (2) sedentary organisms were desirable so that the organisms would reflect the geographical area being studied, (3) the organisms should be numerous, (4) the life span of the organism should last the duration of typical study periods, and preferably longer, (5) the size of the organism should provide enough tissue for convenient analysis, and (6) the organism should be easily collected and easily handled in the laboratory.

Bivalves meet these criteria and have been widely used in studies as indicators of overall water quality and as indicators of pollution by hydrocarbons, pesticides, heavy metals, and radionuclides.[4] Bivalves were first used in general pollution studies estimating species diversity or species prevalence indices.[5,6] (In many polluted aquatic systems, a correlation is seen between increasing pollution and decreasing species diversity. However, diversity studies are difficult to do, are time consuming and often baseline data of normal levels of diversity are not available for comparison.)

Bivalve molluscs have been much more useful as bioaccumulators and monitors of several specific groups of pollutants. Molluscs are filter-feeders, taking the bulk of their nutrients as zooplankton and phytoplankton. This feeding habit exposes bivalves to very large volumes of water leading to bioaccumulation of hydrophobic xenobiotics from the food and from the large quantities of water filtered. For many hydrophobic pollutants,[4,7,8] concentration factors of 10,000-fold in bivalves are common.

The ability of bivalve molluscs to accumulate chlorinated hydrocarbons, petroleum hydrocarbons, radionuclides, and heavy metals (discussed below) has been most notably exploited in two well-known monitoring programs, the Mussel Watch[4]* and the National Pesticide Monitoring Program.[9,10,11]

---

*Technically, true mussels are an anatomical subclassification of the class *Pelecypodia*, and are neither clams nor oysters. However, in the terminology of the commercial fisherman, *mussels* include true mussels, clams, and oysters. It is in the latter sense that the monitoring program was named. Some biologists feel the program might have been more accurately but less evocatively named the Bivalve Watch.

Monitoring Programs Using Bivalves

The Mussel Watch Program was established in 1975, largely due to the efforts of Goldberg.[12] The program workers annually sample clams and oysters from 106 sites on the North American coast; recently, the program has expanded to include European coastal waters. The initial objectives of the program, now achieved, included evaluation of collection procedures and analytical protocols and assessment of the reliability of residue analyses of bivalves. The Mussel Watch and the Pesticide Monitoring Program have created a data base of the levels of various pollutants in bivalves.

Pesticide Accumulation

The National Pesticide Monitoring Program was a broadly based effort to establish baseline levels of pesticides in the environment, including freshwaters and marine waters, human and animal food, air, soil, fish, wildlife and humans.[9] Separate monitoring programs for humans, wildlife, fish, and estuaries (among others) were carried out between 1967 and 1973. The Estuarine Monitoring Program[10] could be considered the parent of the Mussel Watch. This program sampled estuarine molluscs at 170 sites in fifteen United States coastal states assaying routinely for aldrin, dieldrin, p,p'-DDT, p,p'-DDD, p,p'-DDE, endrin, heptachlor, heptachlor epoxide, lindane, methoxychlor, mirex, and toxaphene. The study showed widespread occurrence of DDT and its analogues (63% of all samples), followed by dieldrin (15% occurrence). The other pesticides occurred infrequently and with marked local variation. For instance, toxaphene was infrequently found and then only occurred at low levels, except in a large number of samples from the Georgia coast. The toxaphene in Georgia was found to emanate from a single manufacturing plant.[10]

Especially interesting, the Pesticide Monitoring Program discerned trends in DDT contamination of molluscs in the period 1967–1971. There was a 70 percent decline of this pesticide in eastern oysters over this period and the decline accelerated markedly post-1970. By 1977, a very dramatic decline in pesticide levels had been noted.[11] Bivalves proved to be accurate short-term sentinels of DDT levels since they readily cleanse themselves of accumulated compounds when the level in their environment drops.

Chlorinated Hydrocarbon Accumulation

Like the Pesticide Monitoring Program, the Mussel Watch monitors the tissues of the clams and oysters for chlorinated hydrocarbon pesticides, but also includes in its assays other persistent chlorinated hydrocarbons such as the polychlorinated biphenyls (PCBs). PCB levels found so far by the Mussel Watch vary over a thousand-fold among samples, higher levels generally being associated with coastal waters adjacent to industrialized areas.[4] Several large areas having significantly elevated PCB levels have been identified (San Francisco Bay, San Pedro Harbor, San Diego Harbor, the Boston-to-New York coastal region and St. Augustine, Florida). The wide distribution of bivalves badly contaminated with PCBs probably mirrors the wide distribution of PCB sources in these areas. Only one exceptional hot spot of PCB contamination has been identified and has provisionally been associated with a manufacturer of electrical capacitors, near New Medford, Massachusetts.

Like the Pesticide Monitoring Program, the Mussel Watch is finding strong local variations in the levels of pesticides such as p,p'-DDE and p,p'-DDD. On the West Coast, the program traced at least one case of high contamination to a specific municipal sewage treatment plant outfall associated with DDT residues from a DDT manufacturing plant.[13]

Petroleum Hydrocarbon Accumulation

The Mussel Watch monitors for a broader range of persistent pollutants than did the Pesticide Monitoring Program. In addition to pesticides, petroleum-related hydrocarbons, heavy metals and radionuclides are analyzed. The Mussel Watch Study has shown that it is possible to detect and differentiate petroleum hydrocarbons from naturally occurring hydrocarbons by analysis of indicator compounds such as phenanthrene and dibenzothiophene plus their alkyl-substituted analogues. These aromatics do not naturally occur in bivalves; they apparently come from contamination of the water by oil spills. In general, the program has detected very few samples contaminated by petroleum hydro-carbons (4 out of 83), and, in most of these, the level of contamination was low.

The original Mussel Watch hydrocarbon data has been augmented by certain other reports of the accumulation of hydrocarbons including the polynuclear aromatic hydrocarbon carcinogen benzo(a)pyrene [B(a)P] in bivalves found in polluted harbor waters.[14,15] In this study, the levels of B(a)P were found to vary systematically with the location of the mussel beds relative to the probable sources of hydrocarbon pollution in the harbor.

In another recent report, the mutagenicity of extracts of marine bivalves has been found to correlate qualitatively with the location of mussel beds in polluted versus relatively unpolluted harbors in the United Kingdom.[16] Alcoholic extracts of clams from polluted waters (Plymouth), were several times more mutagenic in *Salmonella* and *Escherichia*-reversion assays, and in *Saccharomyces* gene conversion assays than were extracts from cleaner marine environments (Mumbles, Coswell Bay, and Anglesey, U.K.). The data strongly suggested that the biologically active agents in the clam extracts were frameshift mutagens. Although this study did not include chemical analyses of the clam extracts, it is well known that typical mutagenic polynuclear aromatic hydrocarbons such as B(a)P are frameshift mutagens.

Radionuclide Accumulation

The accumulation of heavy metals and radionuclides by bivalves is probably related to the production of the shell. The Mussel Watch Study found uptake of radionuclides and some heavy metals in both shell and soft parts of bivalves, although bioconcentration factors were much lower than those for hydrophobic organics.

Analyses of radionuclides showed uniform concentrations of ^{239,240}Pu, ^{241}Am and ^{137}Cs in east coast samples and were mostly consistent with fallout as the source.[4] A few anamolous samples were found and, in one case, identified as contaminated by a nuclear fuel facility (Plymouth Bay, Mass.). No important differences in the uptake of the various radionuclides by clams, oysters, or mussels were found. However, the byssal threads of these organisms were found to be enriched in ^{241}Am and ^{239,240}Pu approximately ten times more than the hard or soft parts of the organisms. An interesting insight relating to mechanisms of metal uptake by bivalves was the finding that the majority of the fission-related radionuclides incorporated into bivalves in one Mussel Watch Study appeared to come preferentially from suspended particles rather than from metals in solution.[17] How this finding may bias the interpretation of radionuclide incorporation data is not known.

Heavy Metal Accumulation

In addition to rare earths, bivalves accumulate several heavy metals. Among these are lead, silver, nickel, cadmium, and zinc. The Mussel Watch study did not reveal large areas of serious heavy metal pollution, but many examples of local metal pollution were discerned from the metal content of bivalves. Metal concentrations in bivalves typically varied over a ten-fold range with extremes varying about 100-fold from high to low values. Generalized metal pollution was not found. For example, in one case (San Diego Harbor), the highest value for copper and the lowest value for nickel occurred in the same sample.

From one study of paired samples of clams (*Mytilus edulis*) and oysters (*Crassostrea virginica*) from the same location, the oysters were found to preferentially accumulate silver, zinc, copper, and nickel while the clams preferentially accumulated lead. The relative accumulation of cadmium and mercury by bivalves was not determined in this study. Other studies, however, have reported accumulation of all the metals named above, by various bivalve species.[18-22] Thus, these organisms are potentially useful biomonitors for some kinds of metal pollution, and some species may be particularly well suited for the monitoring of particular metals.

Systematic Factors Affecting Bioaccumulation by Bivalves

The utility of bivalves as bioaccumulators of persistent compounds has led to studies of basic underlying factors affecting compound uptake. A prime determinant of total pollutant accumulation is the lipid content of bivalves. This factor is closely related to the bivalves' sexual cycle, which, in turn, is affected by water temperature.[3] The lipid content of most bivalves will increase before spawning and will decline during and after spawning. For example, in the scallop, increases in the levels of blood lipid and proteins correlated closely with periods of gonadal growth and maturation.[23] Thus, the total amount of a lipophilic compound partitioned into a bivalve may show seasonal variations. Second, different bivalve species have more lipid than others either in total or as a proportion of body weights. Therefore certain species may accumulate more pollutant than others from the same water. Thirdly, stressed animals have been found to lose lipid. For example, the freshwater clam, *Anodonta cygnea,* has been shown to lose a substantial amount of its lipid during prolonged anoxia.[24] The severity and frequency of stress affecting total lipid may be a function of the microenvironment of the bivalve. Stress may also be due to the pollution mirrored in the bivalves' contaminated lipid. Thus, severe pollution may tend to lessen total accumulation of compound and lead to an underestimation of the degree of pollution. The influence of the physical state of a pollutant on uptake has not been adequately studied. The relative efficiency of uptake of soluble versus particulate-adsorbed xenobiotics by bivalves is not known although the study previously cited strongly suggested a preferential uptake of radionuclides from particulate matter rather than from solution. Whether this would also be true of lipophilic pollutants isn't known. Finally, it should be noted that various bivalves are well known to readily take up and to readily *release* hydrophobic compounds, as the concentration of compound varies in their environments. Thus the compound's concentration in the bivalves probably reflects a dynamic time-weighted average of the compounds' concentration in their environment.

To summarize, sexual cycles, stress, and genetic make-up can affect total lipid in bivalves and thereby alter the total accumulation of persistent, lipophilic pollutants. In addition, the specific mechanisms leading to partition of a compound into bivalve lipid are incompletely understood and, hence, it isn't currently possible to predict the effect that the physical state of a compound will have on the extent of its bioaccumulation by bivalves.

The Pathobiology of Bivalves

The Mussel Watch Study found that many of the bivalves in the coastal United States were in poor health. These findings together with a growing body of evidence describing pollution of the coastal environment have stimulated the study of invertebrate pathology. Conferences and symposia have been held to promote this field, including the Symposium on Tumors in Aquatic Animals (Cork, Ireland, 1974), the Symposium on Neoplasms and Related Disorders of Invertebrates and Lower Vertebrate Animals,[25] the Symposium on Neoplasms in Aquatic Animals as Indicators of Environmental Carcinogens,[26] and The Conference on Aquatic Pollutants and Biological Effects with Emphasis on Neoplasia.[27]

Poor water quality has been implicated in a wide variety of pathological changes. Copper has been found to cause degeneration of the stomach of the American oyster.[28] DDT bioconcentrated in the gonad of the oyster has been associated with fewer mature ova, abnormal infiltration of leukocytes in gonads, and hyperplasia of germinal epithelium.[29] Exposure to phenol (1ppm) led to necrosis of the gill and digestive tract epithelium of the hard clam.[30] Finally, there have been several reports associating gonadal tumors in clams with oil spills.[31–36]

Neoplastic Disorders in Bivalves

In addition to the gonadal tumors mentioned above, bivalves frequently exhibit a proliferative disorder of the circulatory system that has been characterized as a malignant neoplasia (but see Mix et al.[37] for a discussion of this classification). Like the gonadal tumors, this condition seemed to be associated with polluted environments, leading to speculation that the pollutants may include genetically active components such as B(a)P that might be directly responsible for the neoplasia. However, Brown and his associates have taken a closer look at this situation and found a correlation between tumors and pollution, but tumors were also found in clams in unpolluted waters.[38] Further study revealed the probable involvement of multiple factors, possibly including unidentified infectious agents.[39] This suggested that the pollution may have been inducing a stress that favored infection, leading ultimately to development of the disease. In a related study, Lowe exposed oysters to DDT, toxaphene, and parathion.[29] The organisms became infected with a fungus that caused lysis of gut, gonad, gill, kidney, and mantle; the unexposed controls were not affected. In this study, a pollution related stress apparently encouraged the development of disease.

On the other hand, a recent Russian study indicates that chemical agents alone can induce tumors in bivalves.[40] The freshwater clam, *Unio pictorum,* when injected with diethylnitrosamine and dimethylnitrosamine, developed tumors in 8 percent to 68 percent of the treated animals; no tumors were seen in controls. Of interest, the latency period ranged from sixty-one to eighty-five days. It may also be recalled that dimethylnitrosamine is formed in the decomposition of sludge in water.[41]

Thus, it is not certain at this time whether the poor state of marine bivalves found by the Mussel Watch is solely the product of chemical pollution of the benthic environment. Pathogenic organisms (perhaps contributed by offshore dumping of sewage sludges) or a combination of pathogens and chemical pollutants may account for much of the diseased benthos.

Corbicula as a monitor of fresh-water quality

The success of the mussel watch study strongly suggested that similar methods might be used to monitor fresh waters. It is often not realized by scientists involved in the evaluation of fresh water quality that clams are widely distributed in the rivers and lakes of the continental United States. Among the species found very widely across the United States is the Asiatic clam, *Corbicula manilensis.*[42] This organism was first introduced into the United States approximately forty years ago on the west coast. Since that time, it has spread across the country and from the southern coasts at least as far north as Lansing, Iowa. It has been suggested that this organism may not tolerate extremely low temperatures, i.e. below 4°C and that this may limit its northern distribution. The success of this species in populating North America freshwaters may be attributed to its tolerance of pollution and to its lack of requirement for a fish host for its larval form. *Corbicula* grows to approximately three centimeters by four centimeters in size and is reported in the literature under several names, *Corbicula manilensis, Corbicula leana* Prime, and *Corbicula fluminea* (Muller), all of which are probably the same species.[43] *Corbicula* is noted for growing in large aggregations in fast flowing streams and water mains where it may impede water flow (fouling). Thus, *Corbicula* has traditionally been classified as a pest clam. Recently *Corbicula* has become a valuable economic resource for commercial bait dealers in the southeast United States.[44]

Viewed as a tool for the assessment of water quality, *Corbicula* offers several advantages.[45] Its tolerance to pollution permits an experimenter to implant it temporarily in cages into streams or effluents to permit it to bioaccumulate any persistent or toxic substances that may be present. Because of its free-living larval form, it may be possible to rear *Corbicula* in the laboratory, removing dependence on naturally occurring beds as a source of organisms. *Corbicula* is known to tolerate removal from water for reasonably long periods of time (it has been successfully received and shipped by bus or plane in insulated boxes without water) thus it is easily handled and transported to study sites. *Corbicula* survives in the aquarium without food for periods of up to six months and thus is easily maintained and is potentially useful for chronic exposures under laboratory conditions.

Experimental

To explore the possibility of using *Corbicula manilensis* as a monitor for freshwater quality, an experiment was carried out in which cages of *Corbicula* were implanted in the Kaskaskia River in central Illinois. The cages were removed at various times over a seventy-two day period. Grab samples of river water and the soft tissues of the clam were analysed for persistent, chlorinated pesticides. Typical results are shown in Figure 11–1. It was found that the clams took up pesticides in the water such as dieldrin, heptachlor, and chlordane. Bioconcentration factors of 1000 to 10000 were observed in the clam fat, relative to the levels in the water. The clams gained weight and deposited shell during the first half of the experiment (data not shown). The experiment will be reported in detail elsewhere.[7]

From this exploratory study the utility of *Corbicula* as a monitor of freshwater quality was demonstrated. The study is continuing, in an attempt to expand the endpoints to include aromatic hydrocarbon accumulation, mutagenic activity in clam extracts, induction of detoxification enzymes, metal accumulation, and pathological study.

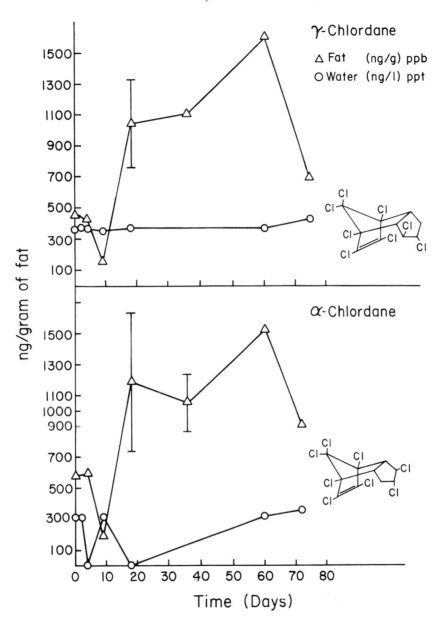

Figure 11–1. Concentration of α- and γ-chlordane in the river water (○) and in the fat of *Corbicula manilensis* (Δ) implanted in the Kaskaskia River. Replicate groups of 50 clams were implanted on day zero and removed for analysis at the indicated times. Pesticide levels in a fraction prepared by florisil and silica gel chromatography of extracted clam fat are depicted.

REFERENCES

1. Goldstein, A., Aronow, L., and Kalman, S. M.: *Principles of Drug Action: The Basis of Pharmacology,* 2nd ed. New York, John Wiley and Sons, Inc., 1975, p. 357–436.

2. Lu, P. Y., and Metcalf, R. L.: Environmental data and biodegradability of benzene derivatives as studies in a model aquatic ecosystem. *Environ Health Perspect, 10:*269, 1975.

3. Phillips, D.: Use of biological indicator organisms to quantitate organo-chlorine pollutants in aquatic environments. A review. *Environ Pollut, 16:*167–230, 1978.

4. Goldberg, E. D., Bowen, V. T., Farrington, J. W., Harvey, G., Martin, J. H., Parker, P. L., Risebrough, R. W., Robertson, W., Schneider, E., and Gamble, E.: The mussel watch. *Environ Contamin, 5:*101–125, 1978.

5. Richardson, R.: Changes in the bottoms and shore fauna of the middle Illinois river and its connecting lakes since 1913–1915 as a result of the increase, southward, of sewage pollution. *Illinois Natural History Survey Bull, 14: 4:*33–77, 1921.

6. Hynes, H.: The use of invertebrates as indicators of river pollution. *Proc Lim Soc Lond, 170:*165–169, 1957.

7. Hartley, D. M., and Johnston, J. B.: Use of the Freshwater Clam *Corbicula manilensis* as a Monitor for Persistent Pesticides. In preparation.

8. Ehrhardt, M., and Heinemann, J.: Petroleum hydrocarbons in oysters from Galveston Bay. *Environ Pollut, 9:*263–282, 1975.

9. Editorial Board: National pesticide monitoring program. *Pest Mon J, 1:*1–21, 1967 and 5:35–71, 1971.

10. Butler, P. A.: Organochlorine residues in estuarine mollusks, 1965–71— National pesticide monitoring program. *Pest Mon J, 6:*238–362, 1973.

11. Butler, P. A., Kennedy, C. D., and Schutzmann, R. A.: Pesticide residues in estuarine mollusks, 1977 versus 1972—National pesticide monitoring program. *Pest Mon J, 12:*99–101, 1978.

12. Goldberg, E. D.: The mussel watch—A first step in global marine monitoring. *Mar Pollut Bull, 6:*111, 1975.

13. Hom, W. J., Risebrough, R. W., Soutar, A., and Young, D. R.: Deposition of DDE and polychlorinated biphenyls in dated sediments of the Santa Barbara Basin. *Science, 184:*1197–1199, 1974.

14. Dunn, B., and Stich, H.: The use of mussels in estimating benzopyrene contamination of the marine environment. *Proceedings Soc Exp Biol Med, 150:*49–51, 1975.

15. Dunn, B., and Stich, H.: Release of the carcinogen benzopyrene from environmentally contaminated mussels. *Bull Environ Contamin and Tox, 15:*398–401, 1976.

16. Parry, J. M.: Monitoring the marine environment for mutagens. *Nature, 264:*538–540, 1971.

17. Goldberg, E. D., Bowen, V. T., Farrington, J. W., Harvey, G., Martin, J. H.,

Parker, P. L., Risebrough, R. W., Robertson, W., Schneider, E. and Gamble, E.: The mussel watch. *Environ Contamin, 5:*101–125, 1978.

18. Davies, I., and Pirie, J.: The mussel *Mytilus edulis* as a bio-assay organism for mercury seawater. *Mar Pollut Bull, 9:*128–132, 1978.

19. Clark, J. H. and Clark, A. N.: On the use of *Corbicula fluminea* as indicators of heavy metal contamination. In Britton, J. C. (Ed.): *Proceedings, First International Corbicula Symposium.* Fort Worth, TX, Texas Christian University Research Foundation, 1979, pp. 153–163.

20. Manly, R., and George, W.: The occurrence of some heavy metals in populations of the freshwater mussel *Anodonta anatine* from the River Thames. *Environ Pollut, 14:*139–154, 1977.

21. Phillips, D.: The common mussel *Mytilus edulis* as an indicator of trace metals in Scandinavian Waters: I. Zinc and cadmium. *Mar Biol (Berl), 43:*283–292, 1977.

22. Phillips, D.: The common mussel *mytilus edulis* as an indicator of trace metals in Scandinavian Waters: II. Lead, Iron and Manganese. *Mar Biol (Berl), 46:*147–156, 1978.

23. Thompson, R.: Blood chemistry, biochemical composition and reproductive cycle in the giant scallop, *Placopecteu magellanicus,* from southeast New Foundland. *J Fisheries Research Board Canada, 34:*2104–2116, 1977.

24. ZS-Nagy, J., and Galli, C.: On the possible role of the unsaturated fatty acids in the anaerobiosis of *Anodonta cygnea* (Mollusca, Pelecypoda). *Acta Biol Acad Sci Hung, 28:*123–132, 1977.

25. Hornburger, F.: *Neoplasms in Aquatic Animals as Indicators of Environmental Carcinogens: Progress in Experimental Tumor Research.* Basel, Switzerland, S. Karger, 1976.

26. Dawe, C., and Harshbarger, J.: *Neoplasms and Related Disorders of Invertebrates and Lower Vertebrate Animals.* Bethesda, MD. Natl. Cancer Inst. Monographs, 1968.

27. Kraybill, H., Dawe, C., Harshbarger, J., and Tardiff, R.: *Aquatic Pollutants and Biological Effects with Emphasis on Neoplasia.* New York, N.Y., Academy of Sciences, 1977.

28. Fujiya, M.: Studies on the effects of copper dissolved in seawater on oysters. *Bull Jnp Soc Sci Fish, 26:*462–468, 1960.

29. Lowe, J., Wilson, P., Rick, A., and Wilson, A.: Chronic exposure of oysters to DDT, toxaphene, and parathion. *Proc Nat Shellfish Assoc, 61:*71–79, 1971.

30. Fries, C. R., and Tripp, M. R.: Cytological damage in *Mercenaria mercenaria* exposed to phenol. In Wolfe, D. A. (Ed.): *Facts and Effects of Petroleum Hydrocarbons in Marine Organisms and Ecosystems.* New York, Pergamon Press, 1976, pp. 174–181.

31. Yevich, P., and Barszcz, C.: Neoplasia in soft-shell clams (*Mya arenaria*) collected from oil impacted sites. *Ann New York Acad Sci, 298:*409–426, 1977.

32. Yevich, P., and Barszcz, C.: Gonadal and hematopoietic neoplasms in *Mya arenaria. Mar Fish Rev, 38:*42–43, 1976.

33. LaRoche, G.: *Biological Effects of Short-term Exposures to Hazardous Materials.*

Proceedings of the 1972 National Conference of Hazardous Material Spills: 199–206, EPA, Office of Hazardous Material, (Washington, D.C.).

34. Barry, M., Yevich, P., and Thayer, N.: Atypical hyperplasia in the soft-shell clam, *Mya arenaria. J Invert Path, 17:*17–27, 1971.

35. Barry, M., and Yevich, P.: Histopathological studies. *Mar Poll Bull, 6:*171–173, 1975.

36. Dow, R.: The ecological, chemical and histopathological evaluation of an oil spill site. *Mar Pollut Bull, 6:*164–173, 1975.

37. Mix, M. C., Pribble, H. J., Riley, R. T., and Tomasovic, S. P.: Neoplastic disease in bivalve mollusks from Oregon estuaries with emphasis on research on proliferative disorders in Yaquina Bay oysters. In Kraybill, H. F., Dawe, C. J., Harshbarger, J. C., and Tardiff, R. G. (Eds.): *Aquatic Pollutants and Biologic Effects with Emphasis on Neoplasia,* New York, N.Y., Academy of Sciences, 1977, pp. 356–373.

38. Brown, R. S., Wolke, R. E., Saila, S. B., and Brown, C. W.: Prevalence of neoplasia in 10 New England populations of the softshell clam (*Mya arenaria*). In Kraybill, H. F., Dawe, C. J., Harshbarger, J. C., and Tardiff, R. G. (Eds.): *Aquatic Pollutants and Biological Effects with Emphasis on Neoplasia.* New York, N.Y. Academy of Sciences, 1977, pp. 522–534.

39. Brown, R. S., Wolke, R. E., Brown, C. W., and Saila, S. B.: Hydrocarbon pollution and the prevalence of neoplasia in New England soft-shell clams (*Mya arenaria*). In *Animals as Monitors of Environmental Pollutants.* Washington, D.C., National Academy of Sciences, 1979 pp. 41–57.

40. Khudoley, V., and Sirenko, O.: Tumor induction by N-nitroso compounds in bivalve mollusks. *Cancer Letters, 4:*346–354, 1978.

41. Kobayashi, M., and Tchan, Y.: Formation of dimethylnitrosamine in polluted environment and the role of photosynthetic bacteria. *Water Res, 12:*199–201, 1978.

42. Morton, B.: Freshwater fouling bivalves. In Britton, J. C. (Ed.): *Proceedings, First International Corbicula Symposium.* Fort Worth, TX, Texas Christian University Research Foundation, 1979, pp. 1–4.

43. Britton, J. C., and Morton, B.: *Corbicula* in North America: The evidence reviewed and evaluated. In Britton, J. C. (Ed.): *Proceedings, First International Corbicula Symposium.* Fort Worth, TX, Texas Christian University Research Foundation, 1979, pp. 250–287.

44. Anonymous: Decline of the asiatic clam in lower Tennessee and Cumberland Rivers. *Spectrum,* Murray State University (Fall), 1980, p. 7.

45. Burress, R. M., and Chandler, J. H., Jr.: Use of the Asiatic Clam, *Corbicula leana* Prime in toxicity tests. *Prog Fish Cult 38:*10, 1976.

Chapter 12

AIR POLLUTION CONTROL AND ITS IMPACT ON HUMAN HEALTH

David L. Swift

INTRODUCTION

Man-made air pollution has long been recognized as a significant environmental problem for urbanizing, technically oriented society. Earlier in this century there occurred several air pollution episodes in Europe and North America that had demonstrable mortality and morbidity effects. As a result of these dramatic occurrences and heightened public consciousness in general, programs were undertaken in the United States to reduce community air pollution. Laws establishing the mechanism for setting standards were passed, and, more recently, the Environmental Protection Agency was established to address and enforce these and other environmental laws. The basis for establishing standards and enforcing controls was stated to be the protection of human health and welfare.

The Clean Air Act provides for a periodic review of the basis of Standards and Control regulations, leaving open the possibility that more strict or more lenient standards may be adopted for specific pollutants or classes of pollutants based on newer evidence. A "Criteria" document, in which evidence of health and welfare effects is discussed, is issued for each pollutant to be controlled accompanied by a document outlining current means for control.

Ambient levels of most criteria pollutants have been significantly reduced in many parts of the United States according to EPA figures. However, in order to achieve compliance nationwide, significant efforts in control are still required. The purpose of this chapter is to present an overview of the technical and economic aspects of air pollution control and consider the probable impact of further controls on human health. Alternate strategies that may be more beneficial to human health will be considered along with their economic impact.

TECHNICAL ASPECTS OF CONTROL

Description of Pollutants and Sources

Air pollution arises from a great variety of sources, chief among which are power generation, transportation, industrial processes, and home heating. Physically, the pollutants include both gaseous and particulate substances. The major gaseous emitted substances are CO, SO_2, NO_X and hydrocarbons. All but CO are capable of atmospheric reaction to produce other gaseous species or particulates. Such substances are known as secondary pollutants, whose control consists of reduction of precursor reactants. Other particulates are generated at the source and are transported in the atmosphere relatively unchanged.

From a control viewpoint, air pollutants are either generated in a contained airflow system, permitting removal by a chemical or physical method, or they are emitted in an uncontained fashion, in which case they are termed *fugitive emissions*. Entirely different concepts of control are appropriate for controllable or fugitive emissions.

Although much innovative effort has been expended to determine relationships between the emission rate and the ambient concentration of an air pollutant, the complexity of possible interactions and loss processes from source to potential receptor make it very difficult to establish such relationship in a general way. Thus, the emission strength and ambient concentration are generally assumed to be linearly related, and, most commonly, a linear rollback approach is used to the estimated degree of emission reduction required to achieve a given ambient level.

Control of Gaseous Pollutants at Source by Air Cleaning

Nonfugitive gaseous emission, e.g. gaseous emission from fossil fuel combustion or contained industrial processes, may be controlled by a number of physical or chemical methods. The general principles that apply to these processes are those applicable to interphase transport in the chemical process industries: these include large interfacial surface areas, equilibrium conditions favoring significant uptake in the capturing phase, and concentration gradients and diffusion controlled layers favoring rapid transport.

A basic difficulty of many gas cleaning applications is that, in contrast to many CPI transport situations, the material to be transported is at a moderately low concentration, often less than 0.1 percent. If more than 90 percent removal is required, it may require elaborate means because of the low transport rates. The scrubbing of SO_2 from coal combustion flue gas is an example of the attempted application of several processes over the last twenty years to achieve more than 90 percent removal and an environmentally acceptable material containing the absorbed or reacted SO_2. The present state of SO_2 scrubbing in flue gases is reviewed by Buonicore.[1] Liquid scrubbing systems producing a marketable product, such as sulfuric acid, have not been successful in the past; similarly, very simple dry scrubbing processes using $NaCO_3/MgO$ injection did not give adequate SO_2 removal. Dry processes involving bag houses or electrostatic precipitators are just now in operation in a few full scale power plants that promise SO_2 removals of 62 to 90 percent for coal sulfur contents from 0.54 to 3.5 percent.[1] From an initial cost and simplicity of operation viewpoint, dry scrubbing coupled with bag house removal appears more attractive than wet scrubbing.

Control of Gaseous Pollutants by Substitution or Modification of Process

Reduction of emmission of gaseous pollutants may also be accomplished by substituting a material whose use automatically assures the desired lower level. The most outstanding single example of this was seen in the early 1970s when most electric utility companies, given the requirement to reduce SO_2 emission, opted to do so with the substitution of low sulfur coal, low sulfur oil, and natural gas for previously used high sulfur coal. Since the supply of low sulfur coal was limited and was in significant demand for metallurgical processes, the conversion to oil fired power plants predominated, and this contributed significantly to increases in the import of crude oil. The economic impact of this increase has been experienced most directly in rising gasoline and fuel oil prices.

Modification of process to reduce emissions has been employed in the cases of NO_x, hydrocarbons, and CO. Alteration in the combustion process in both internal combustion engines and in furnaces have reduced NO_x emissions, but since NO_x generation is associated with increased temperature operation, the thermo-dynamic efficiency in a system of low NO_x emission may be lower than a system achieving very high combustion temperature. Catalytic or combustion afterburning for conversion of CO and hydrocarbons to CO_2 and H_2O have been employed both in internal combustion engines and in smaller stationary sources. Catalytic afterburning is more desirable in most instances (where poisoning is improbable) because of lower temperature operation and absence of fuel requirement for combustion.

Control of Particulates by Air Cleaning

Emission of particulates from controllable sources includes numerous chemical species and physical forms, and the particulate characteristic dimension ("particle size") ranges from 0.005–100 μm. The process most appropriate for air cleaning of a particular emission must be selected based on a proper characterization of the particulates. This includes mean particle size and distribution, number and mass concentration, chemical constituents, phase, and electrical properties in bulk.

Large particulates (particle size $>20\,\mu$m) can readily be collected in sedimentation chambers or large cyclones that are among the most inexpensive air cleaning devices. Particulates with sizes in the range 1 to 20 μ require more expensive means of cleaning including venturi scrubbers, high efficiency cyclones, electrostatic precipitators, spray towers, packed towers, and fibrous filters.

The most difficult particulates to remove with efficiencies approaching 99+ percent are in the size range 0.1 to 1.0 μm. Bag house fabric filter systems are the only practical means of removal for these particulates in large volumetric flow rate sources. These are finding increased application in particulate removal from coal fired power plants because of the less efficient removal of this size range by electrostatic precipitators. Often particulate cleaning devices are used in series, a less efficient precleaner used to collect large particulates and a bag house to achieve the collection of the fine particulates. Particulates smaller than 0.1 μm are transported by Brownian motion and as the particle size approaches 0.01 μm the efficiency for most devices increases; thus, a minimum collection efficiency is observed between 0.1 and 0.5 μm.

Secondary Particulates and Fugitive Emissions

A significant quantity of the airborne particulates in the size range below 1 μm arises by atmospheric gaseous reactions. It has been estimated by the Committee on Particulate Control Technology[2] that approximately 20 percent of the mass of urban particulates are secondary particulates; secondary organics, nitrates, and sulfates. The relative proportion of these three species is, of course, dependent on the relative emission of reactive organic vapors, NO_x, and SO_x, and the conditions for reaction such as temperature, concentration, and electromagnetic radiation. As discussed above, control of these particulates can be achieved by limitation of emission of the precursors, but the present knowledge of the complex chemistry precludes a detailed specification of the significant precursors, especially organic vapors.

Similarly, fugitive emissions are estimated in the normal urban atmosphere to account for as much as 30 percent of the particulate mass.[2] This category of particulates is poorly characterized as to specific source, so that effective control methods depend on a yet-to-be-determined knowledge of the major contributors. Dust suppression has been suggested as a generally applicable method,[1] but has yet to be widely applied.

OVERALL TRENDS OF EMISSIONS
AND AMBIENT LEVELS, 1970-76

Estimates of emission by the U.S. EPA[3] of the major pollutants during the period 1970–76 are shown in Table 12–I. It can be seen that significant decreases during this period occurred for TSP and CO, small decreases for SO_x and HC, and a small increase for NO_x.

Ambient air quality improvements in particulates were reported in[3] New York, Chicago, and Denver. In the New York Air Quality Control Region, it was estimated in 1970 that 60 percent of the population was exposed to particulates at a level above the 75 μg/m^3 primary standard, while in 1976, the ambient data indicated that none of the population was exposed to an annual average

Table 12–I

NATIONAL EMISSIONS ESTIMATES, 10^6 METRIC TONS

Year	TSP	SO_x	NO_x	HC	CO
1970	22.6	29.1	20.4	29.7	99.8
1971	21.4	27.9	21.3	29.3	100.2
1972	20.3	28.8	22.2	29.7	102.0
1973	19.9	29.7	22.9	29.8	98.3
1974	17.5	28.2	22.6	28.6	91.5
1975	14.4	25.9	22.2	26.2	85.9
1976	13.4	26.9	23.0	27.9	87.2

concentration above the 75 $\mu g/m^3$ standard. This was realized by a 30 percent reduction in the TSP annual average. For Chicago and Denver the reductions in ambient TSP concentrations between 1970 and 1976 were 26 percent and 10 percent with decreases of the percentage of population exposed to above 75 $\mu g/m^3$ of 36 percent and 11 percent respectively.

The trends during this period for oxidant and NO_x in the Los Angeles Air Quality Control Region were inconclusive. Similarly, for other areas in California and in the remainder of the country, there were approximately an equal number of measuring stations that showed decreasing and increasing levels of oxidant and NO_x. In 1975, 85 percent of the sites reported oxidant levels above the primary standard of 160 $\mu g/m^3$. Carbon monoxide ambient levels in 202 sites showed decreases from 1970 to 1976 in maximum eight-hour value, 90th percentile of distribution, and percent of time in excess of primary standard exceeded. These data were in agreement with the emission estimates.

Air pollution abatement efforts to the present have been considerable resulting in significant reduction in emissions and ambient levels. However, progress made to date, as discussed above, has been primarily in controllable emissions. Future progress in reducing emission (including fugitive emissions) is likely to be more expensive for an equal percent increment in concentration or emission reduction. It has been estimated by the Council on Economic Quality[4] that in the ten year period from 1978–1987 the total incremental spending on air pollution control will be $278.9 billion, compared to $158.7 billion for compliance with existing water pollution laws, and $40 billion for solid waste, noise, and other environmental quality legislation. It is appropriate to look at the human health consequences of air pollution control proposed, for, as Eisenbud[5] has recently stated "when expenditures are made on so huge a scale, the health effects should be readily identifiable."

HEALTH ASPECTS OF AIR POLLUTION CONTROL

Methodology

Demonstration of the magnitude of human health effects of community air pollution has been undertaken during the past thirty years as the primary basis for air quality standards. Several methods of investigation have been employed involving both nonhuman and human subjects. Acute and chronic exposure studies with various nonhuman animal species have been performed to investigate the dose-response relationship and to elucidate the specific mechanisms of toxicity. In most cases these have been performed at concentrations well above the mean urban concentrations of air pollutants, often at or above the range of concentrations that occur infrequently during episodes.

Two kinds of investigation with humans have been carried out: laboratory exposures of selected human subjects to specific pollutants at low concentrations and epidemiological studies. The latter have been done both for episodic conditions and over lengthy periods of time to detect trends of health that may accompany temporal changes in mean or distributed pollutant concentration. Cross-sectional epidemiological studies have also been undertaken in which morbidity or mortality data are compared to air pollutant exposures of groups of people over a short period of time, usually one to three years. As in all epidemiological studies, it is crucial that other factors (such as smoking) that might produce differences between groups be controlled, and this has been difficult to achieve in many studies.

Studies of Episodes and Their Implications

The acute effect of unusually high levels of pollutants was observed in London in 1952 and 1962. During this period of time, only two pollutants were being monitored, SO_2 and "black smoke," the latter being a parameter related to fine particulates. Since unusual meteorological conditions produced the episode, both pollutants rose in parallel. There was a significant difference in estimated excess deaths between 1952 and 1962 (4000 vs. 700); this was attributed primarily to the observed lower level of smoke whereas the SO_2 level was essentially identical. Subsequent toxicological studies with human and animal subjects have given support to the hypothesis that SO_2 gas alone at concentrations less than 0.5 ppm (1304 $\mu g/m^3$) does not produce effects that merit the level of control proposed.

However, recent studies of atmospheric dynamics[6] suggests that significant conversion of SO_2 to fine sulfate particulates takes place and that these sulfates may be transported over large distances. Studies to date of the toxicity of sulfates at urban ambient concentration (10 to 40 $\mu m/m^3$) do not give evidence of significant effects, but further studies of toxicity and epidemiological studies should be undertaken before a final decision about SO_2 control is made.

Epidemiological Studies at Moderate and Low Levels

Many studies have been carried out to establish relationships between ambient levels of air pollutants and mortality or morbidity. Some of these, such as Lave and Seskin's study[7] of mortality with sulfate and particulates, conclude that a clear relationship exists with moderate air pollution levels, in this instance grouped about a TSP mean value of ~100 $\mu g/m^3$ and an SO_2 mean value of 33 $\mu g/m^3$. Other studies do not report effects observed, for example, the study of Neuberger (8) in Baltimore where TSP, SO_2, and CO levels were collected for a number of census tracts containing middle socioeconomic groups and compared to mortality for a number of specific causes. No correlations were observed from the data that could not be attributed to chance alone. In this case, both TSP and SO_2 exceeded the primary standard in the census tracts with high pollutant levels.

In an attempt to establish thresholds above which health effects occur, EPA carried out a series of epidemiological studies in 1970–71 known as the *CHESS studies*[9]. Some epidemiologists criticized the interpretation and analysis of these studies, and a congressional subcommittee[10] concluded that "technical errors in measurement, unresolved problems in statistical analysis and inconsistency in data in the 1974 CHESS monograph render it useless for determining what precise level of specific pollutants represent a health hazard."

Critical reviews of CHESS and other epidemiological studies that purport to establish the basis for the primary standards of the major pollutants cite reasons similar to the above. A recent review of particulate studies by Holland et al.[11] list a number of difficulties in studies carried out both in Great Britain and United States. They state that "The ultimate test of a causal relationship between particulate pollution and mortality is the demonstration of a reduction in mortality as a result of long-term pollution abatement. The unreality of achieving the pure experimental setting, where other factors such as cigarette smoking are controlled, means that we must look beyond mortality studies for evidence on which to base reliable criteria for levels of pollution which will not affect health."

During the period 1955–1975 in New York City significant decreases in annual average SO_2 were observed; after reaching a peak of 0.24 ppm in 1965 the value fell to 0.04 ppm in the middle 1970s. Analysis of daily mortality in New York City during this period by Schimmel and Murawski[12] show no significant change, an observation consistent with the statement by Holland et al.[11] The inability to observe positive health effects of reduced levels of SO_2 is alluded to by Eisenbud[5] when he states "the subject of health effects of sulfur oxides and particulates is one of the most confusing of the many contemporary environmental issues. The fact that the matter has resulted in such intense debate in the mid-1970s is particularly astonishing because such dramatic reductions in the sulfur dioxide concentrations in many cities in the United States has already taken place, with no indication of any health benefits. This does not imply that such benefits had not occurred."

Acute Laboratory Exposure Studies of Human Subjects

Single pollutant exposure studies of SO_2, sulfate or nitrate particulates, ozone, and nitrogen dioxide have been performed acutely (2–6 hour exposure periods) using human subjects.[13,14] At concentrations significantly greater than the primary annual average standards, changes of pulmonary function can be observed, but only in the case of ozone can measureable effects be observed when the concentration is within three times the standard. Although these studies have been useful in studying the nature of the response to high levels of pollutants, they have not supplied data that can be used to strengthen the case for the primary health standards as they now stand, except perhaps for ozone.

"Inhalable Particles" vs. Black Smoke vs. TSP

As discussed above, particulate measurements in the United States and Great Britain up to the present have been made with two very different methods. The British "Black Smoke" method measures the attenuation of light through a filter paper upon which particulates have been collected. This depends on the physical properties of the particles, but tends to give added weight to particles smaller than 2 μm. The United States method of TSP is a gravimetric method of all particles collected in a high volume sampler onto a filter paper.

It has been argued that TSP may not be a good measure of the health impact of atmospheric particulates since many very large (greater than 15 μm) particles have very little chance of reaching sensitive airway surfaces because they are filtered in the nose or mouth. Consideration is now being given to measure *Inhalable Particles*[15] as a better indicator of potential particulate health impact, these being the particles capable of reaching bronchial or pulmonary surfaces. Like TSP, Inhalable Particles will be gravimetrically determined but will cut off particles greater than 15 μm. Most particulate control measures to date have removed primarily large particles, and this is one possible explanation for the lack of health improvement seen when TSP levels decreased in many United States cities. Unfortunately, the very particulates that are most readily transported to the deep lung are the most costly to remove by the usual control techniques, both because control devices do not efficiently remove them, and because many fine particles are secondary pollutants.

Summary of Health Effects Studies

Most of the epidemiological studies of human health effects reported to date have been for SO_2, sulfates, and suspended particulates (or black smoke in the case of Great Britain). Good evidence for improvement of health has been obtained when levels were reduced from high to moderate, both mortality and reported improvements in symptoms. At levels approaching the twenty-four hour standard for SO_2 and TSP, improvements judged from mortality data cannot be clearly demonstrated if all of the criteria for spurious effects are adhered to.

Fewer studies have been reported for ozone and nitrogen oxides, but human laboratory studies with ozone suggest that effects can be observed (pulmonary functional changes) at levels (0.4 to 0.5 ppm) not much greater than the annual average primary standard (0.15 ppm). As networks to monitor ozone and nitrogen oxides are improved and automobile controls presumably lead to reductions in these pollutants, careful studies to evaluate the possible health impact of these controls should be performed.

ALTERNATIVE APPROACHES TO CONTROL STRATEGY

The present approach to air pollution control consists of primary ambient standards, stationary and mobile source emission standards (existing and new source), provisions to prevent significant deterioration of air quality, and implimentation plans for compliance with standards. The standards, as stated above, have been determined fundamentally to protect health, without regard to cost. Therefore, recent decisions to revert some oil burning power plants to burning coal were justified both on the basis of reducing foreign import of oil and assurance that health would not be affected adversely. Indeed, McCarroll[16] has argued that with appropriate control technology, a significant increase in coal burning can be realized without adverse effects to health.

It has been suggested that in view of the significant reductions that have already been accomplished and the costs to achieve nation-wide compliance for the criteria pollutants that future strategies include cost considerations or the limitation of technology; Others have opted for regulations which will be "technology-forcing." In view of the uncertainties of significant health benefits from further reductions of SO_2 and TSP, some kind of cost-benefit analysis for control, similar to the example of deNevers[17] might be considered. The major problems associated with such analyses are hardly more tractable than those confronting the epidemiologist.

With respect to automobile engine emission, further studies of the toxic mechanisms of ozone and nitrogen oxides at low concentrations are certainly warranted, as are time-series studies of mortality and/or morbidity as urban concentration presumably fall in response to exhaust controls coming into widespread use.

BIBLIOGRAPHY

1. Buonicore, A. J.: Air pollution control. *Chemical Engineering, 87:*81–101, 1980.
2. Committee on Particulate Control Technology: *Controlling Airborne Particles.* Washington, D.C., National Academy of Sciences, 1980.
3. Environmental Protection Agency: *National Air Quality and Emission Trends Report, 1976.* EPA–4501–77–002, December 1977.
4. Council on Economic Quality: *Environmental Quality — 1979.* Washington, D.C., U.S. Government Printing Office.
5. Eisenbud, M.: *Environment, Technology, and Health.* New York, New York University Press, 1978.
6. Subcommittee on Airborne Particles. *Airborne Particles.* Wshington, D.C., National Academy of Sciences, 1977.
7. Lave, L. B., and Seskin, E. P.: *Air Pollution and Human Health.* Baltimore, Johns Hopkins Press, 1977.
8. Neuberger, John S.: *Mortality Impact on Air Pollution in Baltimore City.* Thesis, Johns Hopkins University School of Hygiene and Public Health, Baltimore, 1977.
9. United States Environmental Protection Agency: *Health Consequences of Sulfur Oxides: A Report from CHESS 1970-71.* EPA 650/1–74–004, 1974.
10. U.S. Government, "Report on Joint Hearings on the Conduct of the Environmental Protection Agency's Community Health and Environmental Surveillance System (CHESS) Studies." U.S. House of Representatives, 9 April. Washington D.C., U.S. Government Printing Office, 1976.
11. Holland, W. W., Bennett, A. E., Cameron, I. R., Florey, C. duV., Leeder, S. R., Schilling, R. S. F., Swan, A. V., and Waller, R. E.: Health effects of particulate pollution: Re-appraising the evidence. *Amer J Epidemiology, 110:*525–659, 1979.
12. Schimmel, H. and Murawski, T. J.: The relation of air pollution to mortality. *J Occupational Medicine, 18:*316–333, 1976.
13. Bell, K. A., Linn, W. S., Hazucha, M., Hackney, J. D., and Bates, D. V.: Respiratory effects of exposure to ozone plus sulfur dioxide in Southern Californians and Eastern Canadians. *Am Ind Hygiene J, 38:*696–706, 1977.
14. Andersen, I. B., Lundquist, G. R., Proctor, D. F., and Swift, D. L.: Human response to controlled levels of Inert Dust. *Am Rev Respiratory Disease,*

119:619–627, 1979.

15. Miller, F. J., Gardner, D. E., Graham, J. A., Lee, Jr., R. E., Wilson, W. E., and Bachmann, J. D.: Size considerations for establishing a standard for inhalable particles. *J Air Pollution Control Assoc, 29:*610–615, 1979.

16. McCarroll, J.: Health effects associated with increased use of coal. *J Air Poll Control Assoc, 30:*652–656, 1980.

17. deNevers, N.: Human health effects and air pollution control philosophies. *Lung, 156:*95–107, 1979.

Chapter 13

HEALTH EFFECTS OF
AIRBORNE ENVIRONMENTAL POLLUTANTS

Finis L. Cavender

Introduction

Recent discussions of air pollution have centered on urban air quality as affected by chemical species generated by or related to the combustion of fossil fuels by both stationary and mobile sources. As a direct result of this interest, there are approximately 8,000 air monitoring sites that collect and process approximately 20,000,000 air samples annually.[1] These samples are sent to the National Aerometric Data Bank as a measure of the success of EPA's emission control plans in achieving the National Ambient Air Quality Standard (NAAQS). At present, the NAAQS applies to only six regulated pollutants[2]: (1) particulate matter (TSP); (2) sulfur oxides; (3) carbon monoxide; (4) nitrogen dioxide; (5) photochemical oxidants; and (6) hydrocarbons (nonmethane). This limited atmospheric surveillance does not include large geographic areas or rural populations, nor does it include the environments of the office, the factory, the school, or the home. To consider all potential situations with the same diligence as applied to measuring photochemical oxidants in urban areas would require a seemingly infinite array of monitoring sites with an almost endless list of chemical species to be monitored. It would appear that EPA, in the present NAAQS, is promoting the idea that if one controls the sources of these six air pollutants, one controls most of the deleterious chemical species eminating from mobile or stationary sources.

Health effects range in definition from one extreme, which cites mortality only, to the other extreme, which states that any measurable effect is significant and therefore adverse. Air pollution episodes such as the ones that have occurred in Muese Valley,

London, and Donora have caused increased mortality in the more susceptible subpopulations; however, it is not clear which active agent or agents were responsible or if there was any importance of their sequence of occurrence during the episode. At low levels, it is much more difficult to determine the significance of effects, especially since numerous defense mechanisms are activated in attempts to reduce or prevent respiratory deposition and/or injury.[3] Short-term testing to relatively high levels of pollutants may produce numerous measurable effects including death while long-term exposure to low levels of pollutants may show no measurable effects.[4]

The Respiratory Tract

The respiratory tract is the principle organ system to interface with external environment. For an adult, approximately 10,000 liters of air are inspired in some 21,600 respirations each day. Each breath delivers about 450 cm^3 of air to the respiratory exchange region or alveolar region of the respiratory system. The alveolar surfaces represent an area of about $70m^2$, which is approximately equal to the playing surface of a tennis court.[3] This large surface area efficiently promotes the exchange of oxygen and carbon dioxide; however, with airborne pollutants, this area provides a great potential for injury and disease, especially in view of the fact that the entire blood volume passes through the lung one to five times each minute.[5] The tragedy that can occur is that 10 percent, 20 percent, or even 50 percent of the functional capacity of the respiratory tract may be destroyed before any noticeable change or discomfort is manifested clinically.

Responses to Inhaled Pollutants

The deposition and clearance of airborne pollutants which may include gases, vapors, liquid aerosols, particulate dusts and/or fibers will be discussed according to the physiologic response illicited in the respiratory tract.

Irritants

Irritants can be divided into at least two distinct types. One type, which includes sulfur dioxide and acetic acid, exhibits a biphasic response in the lung. At low concentration, most of these vapors are absorbed in the upper airways and the increase in resistance is due to this upper airway stimulation leading to a reflex bronchial constriction. At higher concentrations, at least some of the vapor reaches the conducting airways and the increase in resistance is proportionally higher. These irritants continue to increase pulmonary resistance over several hours of exposure; however, when the exposure is terminated, the resistance returns to control levels within three hours postexposure. The second type of irritant gas, which includes formaldehyde and formic acid, is more potent and exhibits a unimodel response of increasing resistance with increasing concentration. These irritants usually reach maximum effects within one hour of exposure.

When the exposure is terminated, the resistance decreases markedly, but has not returned to control levels within three hours postexposure.[6,7] Irritant gases like sulfur dioxide can be potentiated by inert aerosols of sodium chloride. Sodium chloride aerosols take up water upon entering the high humidity of the respiratory tract and serve to dissolve sulfur dioxide. Sulfur dioxide now penetrates to the lower respiratory tract dissolved in the aerosol, even at very low concentrations. This sulfur dioxide droplet aerosol behaves like the more potent type irritant gases such as formaldehyde. There is a possibility that some sulfur dioxide is further oxidized to sulfuric acid. All aerosols tested that can dissolve sulfur dioxide upon entering the respiratory tract potentiate the response, while dry aerosols such as ferric oxide do not potentiate the response. The more soluble that sulfur dioxide or another pollutant is in the droplet aerosol, the greater the potentiation.[9,10] Insoluble aerosols do not produce alterations in pulmonary flow resistance in concentrations up to 10 mg/m^3. Thus, they act strictly as a "nuisance dust." Some soluble aerosols, when given alone, e.g. sodium chloride, do not produce alterations in pulmonary resistance except when given with a gaseous irritant, in which case, these soluble aerosols potentiate the response of the irritant gas. Soluble aerosols containing sulfates or amines act as irritant aerosols and cause alterations in pulmonary flow resistance. These aerosols must penetrate the upper airways in order to effect an increase in resistance.[11-13] Therefore, particle size is of extreme importance in eliciting a change in pulmonary resistance.

Inflammation

An inflammatory response in the lung is mediated through thymic dependent (T) lymphocytes. T-lymphocytes are initially of bone marrow origin and play a central role in initiating and mediating delayed immune functions. They attain immunologic maturity under the direction or humoral influence of the thymus.[14] Mature peripheral T-lymphocytes are able to recognize foreign antigens. Specifically, the interaction of T-cells with a foreign antigen results in the synthesis of lymphokines. The association of a foreign antigen, with specifically sensitized T-lymphocytes results in the activation of those cells. Within minutes after interaction with an antigen, alterations in calcium metabolism and membrane morphology occur in T-cells and within hours these cells synthesize new proteins.[15,16] Lymphokines are among these newly synthesized proteins.[17] Lymphokines are instrumental in the recruitment to and activation of macrophages and polymorphonuclear leukocytes (PMN) in the lung. Lymphocyte-derived chemotactic factor (LDCF) attracts macrophages and PMNs to a local tissue site, migration inhibitory factor (MIF) may immobilize these cells at the local site[18] and these cells undergo a process of activation that enhances both their phagocytic and bacterial activities.[19] Activation is probably initiated via the release of C_5 fragments of the complement system. The time course for granulocyte recruitment to airways exposed to endotoxin aerosols shows a peak number of PMNs at four hours in guinea pigs and at six hours in hamsters.[20] Recent studies have shown the increased bactericidal activity to correspond to PMN production of the deadly superoxide radical, O_2^-.[21] The clearance of these phagocytic cells involves their migration to the mucocillary esculator or removal via the lymphatic circulation.

Other Responses

Several other responses can be important, but will not be discussed in detail. These include the coughing, sneezing, mucous production, the speed of ciliary beat, surfactant, biochemical activation, physiological adaptation, vitamin or nutritional status, etc. Oxidant gases may destroy millions of cilia, produce edema by destroying epithelial cells or damaging capillary endothelium, and alter various biochemical and breathing patterns. Severe edema may progress to fibrosis. Many organic dusts initiate a hypersensitivity reaction described as extrinsic allergic alveolitis and repeated exposure precipitates the formation of products that injure cells of the respiratory tract. Dusts as experienced in mines, garages, or milling lead to parenchymal disease called *pneumoconiosis*, which is best characterized as a *swamping* or failure of the self-cleaning mechanisms of the respiratory tract. The most common tumor of the respiratory tract of man is bronchogenic squamous cell carcinoma, which arises from the epithelial cells of the conducting airways. Although twenty years may lapse between initial or known exposure to the causative agent and development of the disease, once the bronchogenic carcinoma is established, extensive invasion and metastases may occur.[3]

Safety Evaluations

The first logical step in the safety evaluation of environmental pollutants is the appropriate standard acute studies. Refinements, improvements, and new testing strategies or techniques are continuously being developed for one pollutant or another, and the new technique may prove to be a consistent, sensitive indicator for that pollutant. Such techniques are readily applied to many pollutants in hope that the improved sensitivity will be universal. Such hopes have been dashed with many promising techniques. Often a technique is a measure of a defense mechanism and while a pollutant may affect the defense mechanism, the reaction may have nothing to do with toxicity unless higher levels of exposure are involved. Even so, techniques such as the measurement of pulmonary resistance and compliance or the breathing rate in mice exposed to pulmonary irritants are very useful in determining which chemical species of a class of compounds may be the most potent. It is not the isolation of the effects on a single defense mechanism but rather the composite response of all mechanisms and the breaching of homeostasis in combination with innate toxicity that determines the adverse health effects of a pollutant.

The process of adaptation can be either beneficial or adverse depending on the circumstances. If one insists on working in the presence of an irritant, eventually, he becomes accustomed to the irritant and the warning system of the irritant response becomes silent unless much higher concentrations are encountered. The dangers of such actions are obvious. Exposure to low levels of photochemical oxidants may cause hemorrhage and edema in the naive animal while continued exposure reveals rapid healing and tolerance with no adverse effects, even with lifetime exposure. Thus, the subtle differences that lead to toxic effects or to increased tolerance are only beginning to be understood. It is important to know as much as possible about the mechanisms of toxic actions and the mechanisms of increased tolerance.

Responsibility

For many environmental settings it may be the balance of these responses and reactions that determine the economic status of entire industries and geographical settings. Opting for a pollutant free atmosphere is as illogical as hiding from the fact that carbon monoxide is life threatening when present in high concentrations. All of the environmental controls imaginable today would not prevent the eruption of Mount St. Helens and the scattering of volcanic ash all over this planet nor will they prevent "natural" death. The directions and decisions we make must evaluate all available facts in making positive decisions that will ensure a safe environment for the next generation. That generation through the iterative process will best be able to make decisions for an even better or safer environment for those that follow. While government and industry and society seem enormously large and unwieldly, it still remains a fact that individual responsibility will effect the greatest results.

REFERENCES

1. Hunt, W. F., Jr., Clark, J. B., and Goranson, S. K.: The Shewhart control chart test: A recommended procedure for screening 24 hour air pollution measurements. *J Air Poll Con Assoc, 28*:508–509, 1978.
2. Ferris, B. G., Jr.: Health effects of exposure to low levels of regulated air pollutants. *J Air Poll Con Assoc, 28*:482–497, 1978.
3. Phalen, R. F., Reischl, P., Faeder, E. J., and Cavender, F. L.: Response of the

respiratory tract to inhaled pollutants. In Willeke, K., (Ed,): *Generation of Aerosols*, Ann Arbor, MI, Ann Arbor Science Publishers, Inc., 1980, pp. 125–139.

4. Cavender, F. L., Sugg, H. W., Cockrell, B. Y., and Busey, W. M.: *Health Effects of Sulfuric Acid Mist.* Presented at the 71st Annual Meeting of the Air Pollution Control Association, Houston, TX, June, 1978.

5. Drew, R. T., and Witschi, H.: Target organ toxicity: Lung introduction. *Environ Health Persp, 16:*1–2, 1976.

6. Amdur, M. O.: The physiological response of guinea pigs to atmospheric pollutants. *Int J Air Poll, 1:*170–183, 1959.

7. Amdur, M. O.: Respiratory absorption data and SO_2 dose-response curves. *Arch Environ Health, 12:*729–732, 1966.

8. Amdur, M. O.: The respiratory response of guinea pigs to histamine aerosol. *Arch Environ Health, 13:*29–37, 1966.

9. Amdur, M. O., and Underhill, D.: The effects of various aerosols on the response of guinea pigs to sulfur dioxide. *Arch Environ Health, 16:*460–468, 1968.

10. McJilton, C. E., Frank, R., and Charlson, R.J.: Influence of relative humidity on functional effects of an inhaled SO_2-aerosol mixture. *Am Rev Resp Dis, 113:*163–168, 1976.

11. Amdur, M. O.: Toxicologic appraisal of particulate matter, oxides of sulfur, and sulfuric acid. *J Air Poll Control Assoc, 19:*638–644, 1969.

12. Amdur, M. O.: The impact of air pollutants on physiologic responses of the respiratory tract. *Proc Am Phil Soc, 114:*3–8, 1970.

13. Amdur, M. O., and Corn, M.: The irritant potency of zinc ammonium sulfate of different particle sizes. *Am Indust Hyg Assoc J, 24:*326–333, 1963.

14. Miller, J. F., and Osoba, D.: Current concepts of the immunological function of the thymus. *Physiol Rev, 47:*437–520, 1967.

15. Allwood, G., Asherson, G. L., Davey, M. J., and Goodford, P. J.: The phytohaemagglutinin. *Immunology, 21:*509–516, 1971.

16. Rosenberg, S. A., and Levy, R.: A rapid assay of cell mediated immunity to soluble antigens based on the stimulation of protein synthesis. *J Immunol, 108:*1080–1087, 1972.

17. Altman, L. C., Snyderman, R., Oppenheim, J. J., and Mergenhagen, S. E.: A human mononuclear leukocyte chemotactic factor: characterization, specificity and kinetics of production by homologous leukocytes. *J Immunol, 110:*801–810, 1973.

18. David, J. R., al-Askari, S., Lawrence, H. S., and Thomas, L.: Delayed hypersensitivity *in vitro.* I. The specificity of inhibition of cell migration by antigens. *J Immunol, 93:*264–273, 1964.

19. Shima, K., Dannenberg, A. M., Jr., and Ando, M.: Macrophage accumulation, division, maturation, and digestive and microbicidal capacities in tuberculous lesions. I. Studies involving their incorporation of tritiated thymidine and their content of lysosomal enzymes and bacilli. *Am J Pathol, 67:*159–180, 1972.

20. Hudson, A. R., Kilburn, K. H., Halprin, G. M., and McKenzie, W. N.: Granulocyte recruitment to airways exposed to endotoxin aerosols. *Am Rev Resp Dis, 115:*89–95, 1977.

21. Salin, M. L., and McCord, J. M.: Free radicals and inflammation: Protection of phagocytosing leukocytes by superoxide dismutase. *J Clin Invest, 56:*1319–1323, 1975.

Chapter 14

EPIDEMIOLOGICAL EVALUATION OF TOXICITY IN STANDARDS DEVELOPMENT

MICHAEL ALAVANJA

INTRODUCTION

Epidemiological research and data have played an important role in the history of regulatory decision-making. This paper will emphasize how epidemiologists must successfully meet several new challenges in the future if they are to continue to have major influence on policy making in occupational health.

According to some public health officials, we are now beginning to reap the bitter with the sweet from the advances of modern technology and industry. For years, most experts in the field of cancer epidemiology believed that the cancer incidence rate in the United States was stable. This is evident from the American Cancer Society's (ACS) 1979 edition of *Cancer Facts and Figures,* which stated that "The overall incidence of cancer decreased slightly in the past 25 years." In the past few months, however, scientists at the National Cancer Institute have released some new evidence that they believe demonstrates a dramatic rise in cancer incidence during the past decade.[1] Although the NCI data have received some criticism, they are convincing enough to have reversed the general consensus. This can be seen in ACS's 1980 edition of *Cancer Facts and Figures,* which states that "The overall incidence of cancer decreased slightly from 1947 to 1970, but has increased between 5 and 10% since 1970."

Marvin Schneiderman, a statistician and former associate director of science policy at NCI, believes that the trend in cancer incidence suggests that industrial exposure may be contributing to the rise in cancer rates and could contribute substantially to the cancer burden in the future. This would be reflected in the so-called occupationally-related cancers, such as respiratory tract, bladder, kidney, and liver cancer, as well as melanoma, lymphoma, and multiple myeloma. Doctor Schneiderman estimates that the rate increased by 25 percent for these occupationally-related cancers from 1969 to 1976.[1]

Doctor Schneiderman's remarks gained additional stature when the leadership of the White House Council on Environmental Quality (CEQ) cited Schneiderman's work in a recent report to the President.[2] The conclusions of this report state the following:

1. the incidence of cancer is increasing;
2. this trend suggests "new or intensifying causal factors";
3. only a small portion of chemical carcinogens have been regulated to date; and
4. exposure to unregulated carcinogens will probably cause the incidence of cancer to continue to rise.

If these statements by the CEQ are accurate, a great deal of additional effort in the areas of environmental toxicology and occupational epidemiology is justified.

Animal studies and, now more then ever, *in vitro* test systems are critical to support environmental regulation because they can provide data in a short time period, allow dose-response curves to be developed, and sometimes give information about a chemical before wide spread human exposure occurs. However, the toxicological problem of translating data derived from animals to humans is likely to remain with us, even when multiple species information is available. Animal studies do not account for the wide social, behavioral, and biological variations in human populations. Such variations can at times be properly ascertained through the use of appropriate epidemiologic techniques that permit direct measurement of responsiveness to toxic agents in humans. The workplace has been a particularly fertile ground for assessing the responsiveness of humans to toxic agents. Before we can detect the health effects associated with low doses of chemicals in the general environment, it is usually beneficial to assess the health effects from high exposure to these same toxic agents in the captive occupational setting.

EPIDEMIOLOGY AND REGULATORY DECISION MAKING

The role that epidemiological research and data have played in regulatory decision making is also most clearly illustrated by focusing on the workplace. Table 14–I and Table 14–II help to illustrate these points by listing the chemicals found in the human environment for which the evidence of carcinogenicity to man was derived from studies that focus on the occupational setting. (Table 14–I and 14–II do not include substances for which the available epidemiological evidence is inadequate.) Workplace environmental standards by OSHA and recommended environmental exposure limits by NIOSH are also listed in Tables 14–I and 14–II, and they represent the product of regulatory decision making that was heavily influenced by these epidemiological studies. Numerous other examples can be given to illustrate this point with other epidemiological end points (e.g., pathologies of reproductive system, CNS, and liver), but these topics are beyond the scope of this paper.

If occupational epidemiologists are to continue to provide public health policy makers with critical data on real people in real environments in the future, five major challenges must be dealt with. Epidemiologists will have to do the following:

1. Assess the hazard of a chemical when limited reliable human exposure data are available;
2. Assess the hazard of specific chemicals among worker populations with multiple exposures;
3. Deal with the phenomenon of component causes of disease;
4. Estimate risk of disease at low exposure levels; and
5. Correct the problem of inadequately documented studies.

ASSESSMENT OF CHEMICAL HAZARD WITH LIMITED RELIABLE EXPOSURE DATA

The problem of trying to assess the hazard of a chemical when limited reliable occupational exposure data are available is widespread. The epidemiologist trying to evaluate latent hazards associated with past exposure to chemical carcinogens must depend

Table 14–I

INORGANIC SUBSTANCES FOR WHICH THERE IS EVIDENCE OF
CARCINOGENICITY TO MAN DERIVED FROM OCCUPATIONAL SETTINGS

Substance	Selected References	Current OSHA Environmental Standard In Air	NIOSH Recommendation for Environmental Exposure Limit
1. Arsenic	Brady et al., 1977, Hernberg, berg, 1977, Lander et al., 1975	10 μg/m³, 8 hr TWA	2 μg As/m³ ceiling (15 minute)
2. Beryllium	Wagoner et al., 1978, Hernberg 1977	2 μg/m³, 8 hr TWA 5 μg/m³, acceptable ceiling 25 μg/m³, maximum ceiling (30 minute)	0.5 μg/m³ (130 minute)
3. Cadmium	Hernberg, 1977 Kolonel, 1976, Lemen et al., 1976	0.1 mg/m³, 8 hr TWA 0.3 mg/m³, ceiling	40 μg Cd/m³ TWA 200 μg Cd/m³ ceiling (15 minute)
4. Chromium	Davies, 1978, Hernberg, 1977, Sunderman, 1976	100 μg/m³ ceiling	1 μg/m³ (Carcinogenic Cr VI) 25 μg/m³ TWA For other Cr(VI), 50 μg/m³ ceiling (15 min.)
5. Hematite	Hernberg, 1977	— —	— —
6. Nickel (organic and compounds)	Hernberg, 1977, Doll et al., 1977, Sunderman, 1976	1 mg/m³ 8 hr TWA	15 μg Ni/m³ TWA
7. Asbestos	Selikoff, 1977, Graham et al., 1977, Peto et al., 1977	2,000,000 fibers/m³ 8 hr TWA; 10,000,000 fibers/m³ ceiling	100,000 fibers/m³ over 5 μ TWA; 500,000 fibers/m³ over 5 microns ceiling

Adapted from P. Cole and F. Merletti: Chemical Agents and Occupational Cancer. *J Environ Pathol Toxicol*, 3:399–417, 1980. Reprinted by permission.

on exposure data gathered when the prevailing philosophy was to measure only infrequently, and then to measure only those environmental components suspected or known to be dangerous. The result is the dearth of environmental data available to epidemiologists today. McDonald et al.,[3] who assessed the effect of chrysotile asbestos exposure on miners and millers, have illustrated one way

Table 14–II

ORGANIC SUBSTANCES FOR WHICH THERE IS EVIDENCE OF
CARCINOGENICITY TO MAN DERIVED FROM OCCUPATIONAL SETTING

Substance	Selected Reference	Current OSHA Environmental Standard in air	NIOSH Recommendation for Occupational Exposure Limit
Coal Soot	Kipling and Waldron, 1976	none	0.1 mg/m³ TWA
Coal Tar	Redmond et al., 1976	none	(cyclohexane fraction)
Petroleum	Decoufle, 1976	(Refined petroleum	
Petroleum Coke		Solvents)	
Wax			
Creosote		500 ppm, 8 hr TWA	350mg/m³ TWA,
Anthracene			1800 mg/m³ ceiling
Paraffin			(15 minute)
Shale Oils			
Mineral Oils			
Auramine	Clayson, 1976,	none	stringent work
Benzidine	Morrison	none	practices and
B-naphthylamine	and Cole, 1976	none	controls, replacement
α-naphthylamine		none	with less toxic
Magnenta		none	materials
4-aminodiphenyl		none	
Mustard gas	Norman, 1975	none	
Vinyl Chloride	Buffler, 1979, Spirtas et al., 1978, Waxweiler et al., 1976	1 ppm 8 hr TWA 5 ppm ceiling (15 minute)	minimum detectable level, 1-ppm ceiling (15 minute)
Bis(chloromethyl) ether	Pasternack et al., 1977, Nelson, 1976,	none	none
Chloromethyl methyl ether	Albert et al., 1975	none	none
Isopropyl oils	IARC, 1977	none	none
Wood dusts	Ironside and Mathews, 1975	none	none
Leather dusts	Anderson et al., 1977, Brinton et al., 1977	none	none

Adapted from P. Cole and F. Merletti: Chemical Agents and Occupational Cancer. *J Envrion Pathol Toxicol,* 3:399–417, 1980. Reprinted by permission.

epidemiologists were able to perform a study when only limited reliable human exposure data were available.

In the eastern portion of Quebec, deposits of chrysotile were first noted in the 1847 Canadian Geological Survey. Within fifty years, this region became one of the world's leading sources of asbestos. McDonald et al. utilized the widespread worker exposure to asbes-

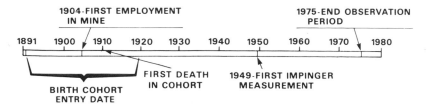

Figure 14–1. Time Line for McDonald's Retrospective Cohort Study in the Asbestos and Thetford Mines in Quebec.

tos in this area as the data base on which to build a comprehensive study on miner and miller exposure to chrysotile asbestos. The principle features of this study are illustrated in Figure 14–1.

The cohort in this study consisted of all 10,939 men and 440 women, born between 1891 and 1920, who had worked for at least a month in the mines and mills of Asbestos and Thetford in Quebec. For all subjects, length of service and estimates of accumulated dust exposure were obtained, including a smoking history for the vast majority. By the end of 1975, 4,463 men and 84 women had died. The time line depicts a rather common characteristic of occupational studies, that being the first exposure occurred years before, in this case 45 years, the first environmental measurements were taken. To overcome this limitation, a tremendous amount of work was directed toward determining the dust exposure for each subject. In essence, 5,783 jobs were identified for each applicable year, and an average dust concentration was estimated in millions of particles per cubic foot (mppcf) from available dust measurements. (Unfortunately, validation of these estimates have not been fully described in the literature.) These estimates were based on more than 4,000 midget impinger dust counts measured between 1949 and 1966. The total accumulated dust exposure for each subject was then summed over a defined period for a defined set of jobs. This is illustrated in Table 14–III.

For a hypothetical worker "A" who spent two years (1904 and 1905) in job category 1 and one year in job category 3 (1906) and two years in job category 6 (1907 and 1908), the accumulated dust exposure would be computed as follows.

$$\text{Accumulated dust exposure for worker A} = \Sigma\ Dj_1y_{1904} + Dj_1y_{1905} + Dj_3y_{1906} + Dj_6y_{1907} + Dj_6y_{1908}$$

Table 14–III

AVERAGE DUST CONCENTRATION (IN MPPCF)
BY JOB CATEGORY AND CALENDAR YEAR

		Calendar Years (y)				
		1904	1905	1906	1907	1908....1975
	1	Dj_1y_{1904}	Dj_1y_{1905}	Dj_1y_{1906}	Dj_1y_{1907}	Dj_1y_{1908}
	2	Dj_2y_{1904}	Dj_2y_{1905}	Dj_2y_{1906}	Dj_2y_{1907}	Dj_2y_{1908}
job (j)	3	Dj_3y_{1904}	Dj_3y_{1905}	Dj_3y_{1906}	Dj_3y_{1907}	Dj_3y_{1908}
Category	4	Dj_4y_{1904}	Dj_4y_{1905}	Dj_4y_{1906}	Dj_4y_{1907}	Dj_4y_{1908}
	5	Dj_5y_{1904}	Dj_5y_{1905}	Dj_5y_{1906}	Dj_5y_{1907}	Dj_5y_{1908}
	6	Dj_6y_{1904}	Dj_6y_{1905}	Dj_6y_{1906}	Dj_6y_{1907}	Dj_6y_{1908}
	.					
	.					
	.					
	j_{5783}					

where D equals the annual average dust concentration for job category j in year y

This procedure to assess accumulated dust exposure was used for each of the 11,379 workers in the cohort.

By utilizing the resultant exposure estimates and the ascertained deaths, McDonald et al.[3] were able to demonstrate a dose-response curve well described by the line:

Relative risk $= 1 + 0.0014$ (mppcf)
of lung cancer mortality

where the exposure variable was dust accumulated to age 45. The linear fit accounted for X^2, with one degree of freedom, of 21.37, leaving only a very low value for deviation from linearity (Figure 14–2).

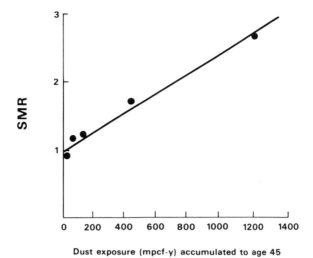

Figure 14–2. Lung Cancer SMRs in relation to dust exposure accumulated to age forty-five.

ASSESSING THE HAZARD OF SPECIFIC CHEMICALS AMONG WORKER POPULATIONS WITH MULTIPLE EXPOSURES

The challenge of assessing the hazard associated with a single chemical in an industry characterized by multiple exposure is well illustrated by a study by Ott et al.[4] In this study, Ott et al.[4] examined the mortality experience of employees with an occupational exposure to styrene in an industrial setting of diverse chemical operations.

The cohort was identified from January census lists of employees for each production or research unit. Entry into the cohort took place from 1937 through 1970. A total of 2,904 persons comprised the cohort. In this occupational environment, many exposures to the chemicals occurred jointly, rather than independently, because of usage patterns. Moreover some workers who changed jobs received different exposures at the different job sites. Thus an exposure categorization approach that reflected both the multiple agents in the environment and the clustering of these agents under certain conditions was needed. The approach Ott et al.[4]

used is depicted in Figure 14–3. In this procedure, Ott et al. did not tally the person years of exposure for an employee until he satisfied the criteria of the category to which he was finally assigned. In a cohort where the individuals changed jobs late in their career, this procedure could result in an underestimation of expected deaths (and thus an overestimation of risk) because person years accumulated prior to satisfying the entry criteria would not be counted. In this cohort, however, the authors stated that this aspect of the study design resulted in less than a 1 percent underestimate in the expected number of deaths because the majority of job

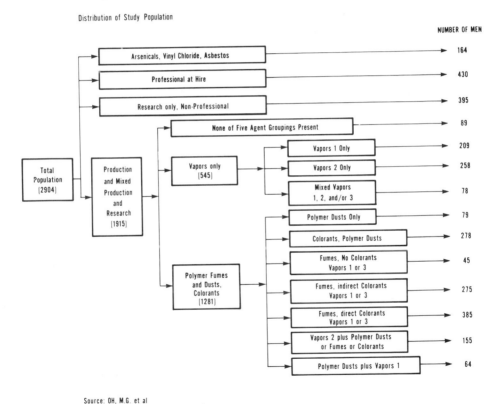

Distribution of Study Population

NUMBER OF MEN

Arsenicals, Vinyl Chloride, Asbestos	164
Professional at Hire	430
Research only, Non-Professional	395
None of Five Agent Groupings Present	89
Vapors 1 Only	209
Vapors 2 Only	258
Mixed Vapors 1, 2, and/or 3	78
Polymer Dusts Only	79
Colorants, Polymer Dusts	278
Fumes, No Colorants Vapors 1 or 3	45
Fumes, indirect Colorants Vapors 1 or 3	275
Fumes, direct Colorants Vapors 1 or 3	385
Vapors 2 plus Polymer Dusts or Fumes or Colorants	155
Polymer Dusts plus Vapors 1	64

Total Population (2904)

Production and Mixed Production and Research (1915)

Vapors only (545)

Polymer Fumes and Dusts, Colorants (1281)

Source: OH, M.G. et al

Figure 14–3. Distribution of study population according to 14 mutually exclusive groups based on environmental and socioeconomic considerations. From M. G. Ott et al.: A Mortality Survey of Employees Engaged in the Development or Manufacture of Styrene Based Products. *JOM, 22(7)*:445–460, 1980. Courtesy of *Journal of Occupational Medicine.*

changes occurred early in the worker's careers.

An additional problem that may result from utilizing this technique may be illustrated by the situation in which workers are exposed to a single chemical that was sufficient to induce disease and later are reassigned to jobs where additional exposures occurred. Under these circumstances, cases would be erroneously ascribed to the multiple exposure category and the elevated observed risk would be magnified by counting only the person years accumulated in the multiple exposure category.

The results of the Ott et al.[4] investigation suggest that employees who had exposure to polymer extrusion fumes, solvents, and colorants had increased risk to lymphatic leukemia (Table 14–IV) but were not at increased risk when exposure to the chemicals was considered individually rather than jointly.

This technique, if used with proper regard to the potential biases, may be used to characterize exposure in other epidemiological investigations involving complex work environments and thereby help meet the challenge of assessing the hazard of specific chemicals among worker populations with multiple exposures.

COMPONENT CAUSES OF DISEASE

A third challenge to the occupational epidemiologist is to adequately address the phenomenon of component causes of disease in occupational studies and to transmit the implications of this phenomenon to other occupational health professionals. The concept of more than one "cause" for a particular disease is straightforward (for example arsenic, chromium, iron oxide, nickel, and asbestos are all inorganic causal agents that can result in lung cancer in humans). However, it is often difficult to deal with the concept of component causes of disease. Most "causes" of disease in the health field are components of sufficient causes, but are not sufficient in themselves. Drinking water contaminated with vibrio cholera is not sufficient to produce cholera, as demonstrated by an attack rate for individuals that drink this water that is rarely 100 percent. Nor is lung cancer mortality inevitable for heavy smokers of cigarettes. The concept of component causes of disease may have best been explained by Kenneth Rothman of Harvard Uni-

Table 14–IV

OBSERVED AND EXPECTED DEATHS DUE TO ALL
CAUSES BY EXPOSURE CATEGORY, 1940–1975

Exposure Category	Total Obs Exp[*]
Mutually exclusive groups	
Research only	44/53.5
None of agents present	13/8.9
Vapors 1 only	23/17.6
Vapors 2 only	53/54.3
Mixed vapors 1, 2 or 3 only, or all	24/15.5[†]
Extr/PD-A only	8/9.2
Colorants-B only	19/19.1
Extr/PD-B, vapors 1 or 3, no colorants	1/2.4
Extr/PD-B, vapors 1 or 3, colorants-A	21/22.4
Extr/PD-B, vapors 1 or 3, colorants-B	54/52.3
Mixed vapors 2 plus Extr/PD-A or B	14/24.0
Vapors 1 plus Extr/PD-A	8/7.8
Agent groupings taken individually	
(same persons may be in multiple groups)	
Vapors 1-A	87/88.3
Vapors 1-B	57/55.4
Vapors 2-A	91/94.4
Vapors 3-A	1/2.4
Vapors 3-B	2/3.0
Extr/PD-A	38/45.6
Extr/PD-B	87/94.8
Colorants-A	22/26.5
Colorants-B	87/95.1

Adapted from Ott et al.: A Mortality Survey of Employees Engaged in the Development or Manufacture of Styrene-Based Products.
JOM, 22:445–460, 1980.

[*]Expected deaths were calculated based on interval-specific SMRs from an internal company comparison population.
[†]p $\leq$ 0.05 based on Poisson distribution.

versity.[5]

In a paper published in 1976, Rothman illustrated the concept by a series of circles representing a set of sufficient causes for one disease (Figure 14–4).

In this depiction, factors A,B,C,D, and E must at some point be present in order to cause a disease by the mechanism of sufficient cause I. Likewise A,B,F,G,H, must be present for sufficient cause

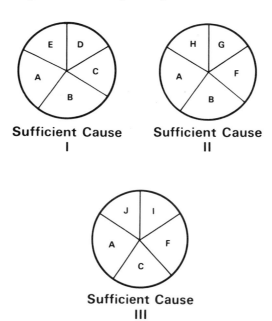

Figure 14–4. Conceptual Scheme for the Causes of a Hypothetical Disease. From K. J. Rothman: Causes, *Am J Epidemiol*, *104*:587–592, 1976. Courtesy of the American Journal of Epidemiology.

II, and A,C,F,I,J must be present for sufficient cause III.

This model helps demonstrate that risk factors for disease are often not intrinsically strong or weak. A component cause that requires other components with low prevalence is thereby seen as a weak component cause. On the other hand, a component cause dependent on other component causes that are ubiquitous seems to be a strong component cause.

Consider the following greatly simplified example. In a society where there was ubiquitous, but unrecognized exposure to a cancer-promoting agent, a rare occupational exposure to an initiating agent would appear to demonstrate that the agent was a "strong" risk factor for cancer. But in a society where there was rare exposure to that same cancer-promoting agent, an occupational exposure to the same initiating agent would appear to demonstrate that the agent was a "weak" risk factor.

The concept of component causes of disease is illustrated by the epidemiological data now available indicating that dietary ingredients are, in some manner, related to cancer. The vitamins that have been associated with nutritional effects on cancer include vitamin A and vitamin C (ascorbic acid). Other epidemiologic studies have associated the quality and quantity of dietary fat with certain forms of cancer, particularly of the colon and breast. Well controlled animal studies have tended to support these epidemiologic findings. The point is that most factors related to nutrition and carcinogenesis are not carcinogens, but are modifying factors, that is, component causes of disease. These observations would suggest that these causal associations are complex and require further investigation as to the mechanisms involved.

Fortunately for occupational epidemiologists, identification of all the components of a given sufficient cause is unnecessary for prevention, because blocking the causal role of only one component of a sufficient cause will make the joint action of the other components insufficient, thereby preventing the effect by that sufficient cause. Yet, sufficient attention to the challenge of dealing with the concept of component causes of disease is vital to the proper interpretation of epidemiologic data and the proper formulation of occupational health policy.

ESTIMATING RISK OF DISEASE AT
LOW EXPOSURE LEVELS

A fourth challenge that epidemiologists together with toxicologists and biostatisticians must meet is the challenge of estimating the risk of disease at low exposure levels. The Supreme Court, by a vote of five to four in the benzene decision,[6] upheld the ruling by the Court of Appeals which stated that the Occupational Safety and Health Administration (OSHA) exceeded its authority when it proposed a benzene standard of 1 ppm and failed to show that the standard was reasonably necessary or appropriate.

OSHA's case for the benzene standard was ruled inadequate because OSHA neither demonstrated a leukemogenic risk at the existing limit of 10 ppm nor quantified the health benefit that would result from reducing the limit from 10 ppm to 1 ppm. Moreover, the Court found that the 1 ppm level was not established on the basis of empirical evidence but on a "series of assumptions," most notably OSHA's cancer policy. The majority decision contended that the government's case for a more stringent standard was weak because the case relied on an "assumption" that the risk of leukemia will decrease as exposure levels decrease without the support of a dose-response curve. Clearly the Supreme Court's decision will make the government's job of regulating toxic substances even more complex than in the past. In order to meet this challenge, health scientists should feel compelled to develop methods to estimate risk of disease at low exposure levels where no direct evidence is available. This task of risk assessment has already been started, but methods of increased sophistication that realistically consider the chemical and biological mechanisms at work will be needed.

PROPER DOCUMENTATION OF STUDY METHODS AND RESULTS

The fifth and final issue is unlike the preceding four issues. It is not of theoretical importance, but is of great practical importance to public health policy makers. The issue is the need to properly document study methods and results.

Frequently, the information supplied by the author of a paper is inadequate to make an objective evaluation and interpretation of that epidemiological study. Gaps in the documentation of these studies have often led to conflicting decisions by agencies with related responsibilities. In order to correct this situation the members of the Interagency Regulatory Liaison Group (IRLG) have recently proposed a set of guidelines for reporting epidemiological studies. The agencies in IRLG include the Environmental Protection Agency (EPA), the Consumer Product Safety Commission (CPSC), the Food and Drug Administration (FDA), the Occupational Safety and Health Administration (OSHA), and the Food Safety and Quality Service of the Department of Agriculture (NIOSH is not a regulatory agency and is therefore a participant in IRLG meetings but a nonvoting member). The proposed guidelines are intended to promote full documentation of submitted research and thereby permit the objective evaluation of study results and conclusions, which in turn will further enhance the role of epidemiology in the regulatory process.

More complete documentation will be particularly helpful when a number of studies suggest divergent conclusions. The weight given to the findings of any individual study will be made on a more rational basis. Weighting will depend on the scientific excellence of the study that will be apparent because of the more fully documented protocol and results described in the report. Seven specific areas of documentation mentioned by the IRLG are summarized here.

1. *Background and Objective*

   The pertinent scientific background leading to the study as well as the study's sponsorship and sources of funding should be given. The objective should be clearly stated.

2. *Study Design*

   The study design should be described and justified in relation to the stated objectives of the study. Limitations of the study design with regard to the stated objectives should be described in detail.

3. *Study Subjects*

   A description of the population from which study subjects were selected and the method of selection should be given.

4. *Comparison Subjects*

   The appropriateness and possible limitations of the group(s) selected for comparison should be discussed.

5. *Data Collection Procedures*

   The procedures by which data are collected will influence the interpretation of epidemiologic studies, so a full discussion of data collection procedures should be included.

6. *Analytic Methods and Statistical Procedures*

   A description should be given of the procedures and analytic method used to estimate risk or to test specific hypotheses.

7. *Interpretation, Limitations, and Inferences*

   Interpretation of the study results should be given in relation to the stated objectives of the study. Special consideration should be given to limitations of the data and the specific methods of analysis used for the study. Interpretation of the study results and inferences drawn from that interpretation should be supported by discussion of probable bias, biological plausibility, and consistency in relation to other studies— both human and experimental.

It is hoped that these guidelines and the other efforts by epidemiologists outlined in this chapter will help make the regulatory process an even more effective tool toward promoting public health in the future.

REFERENCES

1. Schneiderman, M. A.: *What's Happening to Cancer in Our Advanced Industrial Society?* Presented at the Conference on Epidemiological Methods for Occupational and Environmental Health, Washington D.C., December 3–5, 1979.
2. Toxic Substances Strategy Committee: *Toxic Chemicals and Public Protection, A Report to the President.* Washington, D.C., U.S. Government Printing Office, May, 1980.
3. McDonald, J. C., Liddell, F. D. K., Gibbs, G. W., Eyssen, G. E., and McDonald, A. D.: Dust exposure and mortality in Chrysotile mining, 1910–75. *Br J Ind Med, 37:*11–24, 1980.
4. Ott, M. G., Kolesar, R. C., Scharnweber, H. C., Schneider, E. J., and Venable, J. R.: A mortality survey of employees engaged in the development or manufacture of styrene based products. *JOM, 22:*415–560, 1980.
5. Rothman, K. J.: Causes. *Am J Epidemiol, 104:*587–592, 1976.
6. Industrial Union Dept, AFL-CIO v. American Petroleum Institute et al. and Ray Marshall, Secretary of Labor. American Petroleum Institute et al. Supreme Court of the United States, July 2, 1980, 100 SCt 2844.
7. Interagency Regulatory Liaison Group: Epidemiology work group— Availability of draft guidelines. *Federal Register, 44:*67232, Nov. 23, 1979.

INDEX

237